Parkinson's Humor

Funny Stories about My Life

with Parkinson's Disease

By Beverly Ribaudo

ISBN-13:978-1478325840

ISBN-10:1478325844

I want to thank the following people:

My Wonderful Husband, who always takes such good care of me. I love you very much. Thanks for all your help in editing the original blog stories and for encouraging me to keep spreading the laughter.

My Parkie friends: Karyn Spilberg, whose suggestion to write a blog was the start of all this fun and Steve and Linda, for running the Parkinson's Chat Room where I met so many wonderful new friends.

My friends Penny and George, who helped edit this book.

The Yuma Camera Club, for helping me to become a better photographer.

My new friends at Write on the Edge, who explained how to self-publish my book so I can share it with you.

To Dad and Mom, you taught me how to laugh at life's ups and downs and keep smiling.

Thank you for reading my book, I hope you will learn more about Parkinson's.

Table of Contents

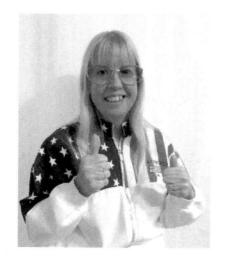

Things Happen for a Reason

In March of 2011, I read a Letter to the Editor in the *Yuma Sun*, our local paper. The letter writer had Parkinson's and he was inviting the public to attend an upcoming Parkinson's disease (PD) seminar.

I had been diagnosed (at age 47) with Parkinson's on August 30, 2007. In the three and a half years since, I'd only met one other person with Parkinson's, and hadn't really learned much about my disease. I saved the paper and asked my Wonderful Husband if he wanted to go to the seminar with me. He reluctantly said yes. He's very shy and doesn't like medical stuff so, being in a room full of strangers and listening to doctors speak, would be just slightly more appealing than going to a dentist for a root canal.

We went to the seminar and I was amazed at how much I learned in those two days. I learned people with Parkinson's have a nickname; Parkies. I found out there were online chat rooms where people with Parkinson's could talk to each other. I met Greg (the letter writer from the paper) and he invited me to join the local support group. I met other people with Parkinson's. Oh, I also learned some stuff about my disease.

Greg's Letter to the Editor would change my life and it almost didn't happen. You see, I usually skip the "Letters to the Editor" section of the paper, but for some reason, on that day, I didn't.

Chatting in the Night

I was up very early one morning (a common occurrence for me since I began taking medicines for my Parkinson's) and just wanted to talk to someone. Sure, I could have woken up my Wonderful Husband, but he looked so peaceful, sleeping soundly, that I just couldn't do it. I played solitaire on the computer for a while, but I really wanted to talk to someone, anyone.

I went online and typed Parkinson's chat room in the Google search box; I selected a listing, logged in and hit the jackpot. I wasn't alone! Also logged in were Mary from Mississippi, Andrew from Australia and Karen from England. You see, when it's 4 am in Yuma, Arizona, it is 6 am at Mary's, noon in England and 10 pm the next day in Australia.

They made me feel very welcome and we chatted about all kinds of things (some of it even related to Parkinson's); we shared stories and then Andrew showed us his pet python snake on his web cam. Now, most girls would have logged out, but I am a bit of a tomboy and I'm not afraid of snakes, my late stepson, Mark, had snakes and my grandson, Travis, does also.

In the months after, I met many more Parkies from the U.S.A. and around the world and as we chatted in the wee hours, I told them funny stories and I became known as Yuma Bev.

8

Why Yuma Bev? I am lazy, pure and simple; it was just plain laziness on my part. I didn't want to keep typing Yuma when asked where I was from by new people I met in the Parkinson's chat room. So one day I added Yuma in front of Bev when I logged in. It stuck and is now how I am known around the world!

Karyn, a Parkie from Australia, was writing a blog about getting Deep Brain Stimulation (DBS) surgery, a procedure to relieve PD symptoms, and she is the one who inspired me to share my funny stories in a blog.

So, Parkinson's Humor was born. I have to admit that when I wrote the first story (I Am Special) at 4 am on Sunday, July 17, 2011, I did not think anyone would read it, except my Wonderful Husband. It was nice to be proved wrong.

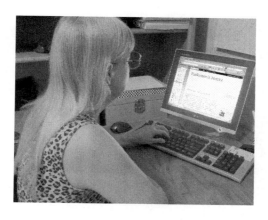

YumaBev blogging

I Am Special

I have Young Onset Parkinson's disease (YOPD), also known as early onset. What does Young Onset mean, exactly? It means that instead of waiting until my late sixties to get this disease, I was precocious and got it in my thirties. This makes me special, just like Michael J. Fox, but without his bank balance. It also means I didn't have to wait until 62 to collect Social Security or 65 to get on Medicare. I get both now, thanks to Parkinson's. Of course, the check I get is not near what I made when I could still work, but I don't have to commute or wear high heels.

I may be special, but I am not rare. For a while, I thought Mr. Fox and I were the only Young Onsets out there. I was wrong. I have since found quite a few other precocious people, some in their early twenties.

A sense of humor is a requirement when you have Parkinson's. Not only is it a good idea to be able to laugh at your predicament, but laughter helps your brain produce more dopamine, which is the stuff we are lacking and causes all of our weird symptoms.

I was never, what I would call, normal. I was always small for my age and a couple years ahead of the rest of the class in school. My Mother used to say I had "an old soul" and maybe it's my "old soul" that got the Parkinson's.

Darn! Maybe I am not special after all.

My Definition of Parkinson's

If you read the medical definition of Parkinson's, it sounds like a drawn out oxymoron. "Parkinson's disease is a degenerative neurological disease characterized by involuntary movements and lack of movement." What?

I think of Parkinson's as a communications problem. My brain is saying one thing and my body is doing something else.

Parkinson's reminds me of a boy I knew in high school. He had an older car, a fixer upper. This car seemed to be possessed. One day, he would turn on the radio and the headlights would come on. The next day, he would turn on the wipers and the horn would blow or the turn signals would come on. It seemed like gremlins were re-wiring the car while he slept. It drove him crazy. He never knew what was going to happen when he got in the car to drive to school in the morning. Every weekend he would search under the hood for the problem and find nothing. No blown fuses, no burned wires, everything looked kosher.

Then one day he saw some seeds on the floorboard. That's strange, he thought. The car was closed up tight and locked. The next day he found more. He did some digging and found out a squirrel had been nesting inside his dash. Scrambling around in the night and sneaking out in the morning. This was the cause of his electrical problems: seeds, twigs, and pieces of trash, all hidden behind the dash.

11

Parkinson's is a lot like that squirrel in the dash, messing around, so you don't know what will happen when you try to blow your horn!

I Re-write the Songs

I have a knack for re-writing the words to songs, it's easy for me and I have been doing it since my teens. I hear a song and new words pop into my head immediately. I admit that the words I came up with years ago were not always designed for family audiences, but hey, I was a teenager.

I kept these lyrics to myself, singing only to the radio when I was alone. You see, I know I can't sing. I entered a school talent show when I was in sixth grade and my teacher took me aside and gently said "Beverly, I am sorry, but you sang every note off-key." and she was right, I couldn't carry a tune, not even in a bucket.

That didn't stop me from composing new parodies, like the one I wrote a few years ago, about RVers (people who are living in a Recreational Vehicle, like a motor home or camper) heading back home after spending the winter in Yuma. I was living in an RV Park at the time and overheard the manager say "Another one left the park today." and that was all it took. I went home and wrote Another One Leaves the Park to the tune of *Another One Bites the Dust* by Queen. I surprised everyone, including myself, by showing up at the community hall for karaoke night and singing it. It was the first time I had sang in public since the sixth grade and no one booed; they LAUGHED and joined me in singing the chorus before the song was over. If I had a perfect voice, it wouldn't have been as funny.

13

Since then, I am unstoppable; I write songs about everything and anything, most of them funny. Sometimes all it takes is a comment or a saying on a t-shirt, to inspire a song. I've written songs for WWII Veterans, Birthdays, Anniversaries and a song about Angels (one of the few serious songs I've done). I've even written songs about Parkinson's. I use karaoke tunes for the melodies, but I copyright my lyrics (I submit them as poems, which is what lyrics really are).

Since I cannot upload the songs by themselves to my website, I make music videos of them and upload them to YouTube and so far, the owner's of the music haven't objected. So I keep creating them and people keep listening and hopefully laughing.

I wonder what Mrs. Serles (my sixth grade teacher) would think?

PS I will tell you how to find all my YouTube videos at the end of this book (including Another One Leaves the Park).

Okay, Seriously, What is Parkinson's?

Parkinson's disease is caused by the death of little neurons in an area of your brain called the substantia nigra (black substance), which is located deep inside and somewhere above the spinal cord. These little gray cells, as Hercule Poirot would call them, make a chemical called dopamine.

Dopamine helps your brain send messages to movement related parts of your body. As these neurons die off, less dopamine is produced and the messages get garbled. These garbled messages cause a myriad of symptoms, ranging from twitching pinkie fingers to becoming stiff and rigid like a mummy and can change from hour to hour and day to day, but progressively becoming worse as more neurons go to gray cell heaven.

Each and every Parkie can have different symptoms. Most start with just symptoms on one side of their bodies. Mine was my right hand, very bad for a right-handed person. If I had been a lefty, I might not have even noticed for a while. Most notice a shaking or tremor as the first sign, others never get tremors and just feel like their limbs got filled with concrete when they weren't looking; others have dexterity problems. My first symptom was the inability to double click my computer mouse with my right index finger, even though I had done it the day before with no problems. These discrepancies can make diagnosis very difficult.

There is no test for Parkinson's; yet. They rule out everything else and then make an educated guess. In my case, it took over eight years before someone guessed right. Another Young Onset I met online got the right guess the day after she noticed something amiss.

The average time to diagnosis for us youngsters seems to be a couple of years. The doctors are looking for other things, not an "old persons" disease and sometimes tell us that it's all in our head. That part they are actually right about; it IS all in our head, it's just not imagined.

The Thrift Store Queen

I love to go shopping at thrift stores (resale shops run by charities). My friends call me the Thrift Store Queen. I look for costumes for my various music skits, t-shirts with funny sayings and items to decorate our gravel yard. I rarely spend over $1 per item and often purchase nothing, but I enjoy the looking around.

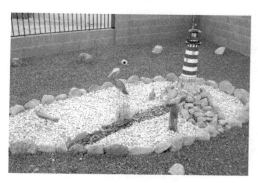

Our decorated gravel yard

One day I saw something I could not resist. A sequin gown! Now, I need a sequin gown about as much as I need Parkinson's. I have no place to wear one, but I have always wanted one. This one was royal blue, the exact color I've always wanted. I took it into the dressing room to try it on. I could fantasize for a little while, couldn't I? I mean, what could it hurt?

It seemed the right size, but it had no zipper or buttons. I tried to put it on. I got my head and both arms through and promptly got stuck. Completely stuck! It wouldn't

17

come off or go on. I was stuck and all alone, having left my Wonderful Husband at home. He normally comes with me if I am shopping for clothes.

So, there I was, a 49-year old woman with granny type sneakers on my feet, stuck in a dressing room with a sequin gown half on. I didn't know what to do! All the nearby voices seemed to be teenagers and I wasn't going to embarrass myself in front of a teen. So, I kept wriggling and got stuck worse.

Finally, I heard a familiar voice, a close friend, who is also a thrift store diva. I called out her name and she helped me get the gown off. We had a good laugh and I treated her to dessert at a restaurant nearby. Then she said, "I bet you are supposed to step into that gown, not put it on over your head." So we went back and I tried it again and it fit, perfectly, though I still needed help. So, I blew my budget and spent the $6 to buy it.

I took the gown to the best alterations place in town and asked the owner if she could put a zipper in it. She took a close look at it and said "No way, this is custom made; one mistake and the whole gown will unravel." She asked how much I paid for the gown, and I said "Six." She said "$6000, that's a great price!" I left her shop, smiling from ear to ear!

A few months later, in October of 2009, I treated my Wonderful Husband to a cruise for his birthday. My Wonderful Husband and the Captain shared the same first name and both had relatives in the same town in Italy, so I got my picture taken with the two best looking men on the ship, wearing my blue sequin gown!

It turns out that I really, really did NEED a sequin gown after all.

My Wonderful Husband tells everyone that my gown cost $606 ($6 for the gown and $600 for the cruise, so I could wear it.)

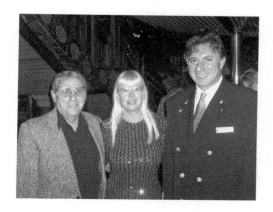

Wonderful Husband, Bev, Captain

What Does Parkinson's Feel Like?

People often ask me that question and I have thought about it a lot over the years. Probably the easiest symptom to duplicate is the lack of dexterity in my fingers and hand. Want to give it a try? See what it feels like? Okay, go dig out your winter gloves. Got them? Good. Now, let's set up some tests for you. Grab a deck of cards or a stack of dollar bills. Are you wearing anything with buttons? If not, grab a shirt out of the closet. Ready?

Put the wrong glove on backwards on your dominant hand. Now, try to deal the cards or count your dollar bills. Having trouble? Now try to button or unbutton those buttons. Fun, isn't it? That's what my right hand feels like 60% of the time. The rest of the time, it feels like I have an invisible glove on, just not the wrong one backwards. So, now you can understand why I could no longer be a bank teller, however, I excel at the children's card game known as 52 pick up.

There is no pain in my hand or fingers like you get with arthritis. There is no tingling, numbness, loss of strength or feeling. The fingers just won't cooperate with my brain. If I need to open a jar of pickles, my right hand is the one I use, IF I can get it to grasp the lid. Cutting steak is also difficult, trying to coordinate both pushing down and moving back and forth.

20

So, we Parkies adapt. My Wonderful Husband cuts my steak when my fingers won't. I donated most of my shirts with buttons to the Salvation Army or now wear them over tank tops and just tie the tails in a knot at my waist and skip the buttons. It works. for me, and looks fashionable, too. Plus it was fun shopping for the right color tank tops to wear under my favorite shirts.

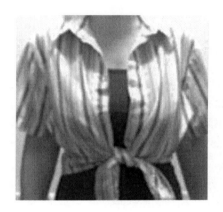

Aunt Cynnie

Parkinson's will sneak up on you, if you aren't paying attention. Sure, I noticed the tremors, but the rigidity and slowness, not so much. The first time I noticed how slowly I moved was in 2004; on a cruise ship filled with seniors and I was completely shocked. My Wonderful Husband (who is twenty years older than me) was taking the stairs two at a time and then I noticed that almost everyone was walking faster than me, even the folks with walkers and canes.

The real kicker came in 2006, when I went to visit my Aunt Cynnie who lived by herself in an upstairs apartment. I hadn't seen her in years and yet, when my Wonderful Husband and I got to her door, she asked me if I could make it up the stairs. Somehow she knew those thirteen stairs would give me trouble. So, there I was 46-years old and being helped up the steps by a tiny and almost blind 94-year old woman. We joked about it every phone call after that. She lived to be 97 and could still take those stairs better than I could.

Aunt Cynnie was my Mom's oldest sister, the first born in her family. My Mom was the youngest and there were two in between; George and Belle. I'm not sure what order they came in. Aunt Cynnie married late, at age 28, and became a widow twenty years later, when her husband died of a heart attack. They never had any children, but George had four, Belle had one and my Mom had five, so Aunt Cynnie had plenty of nieces and nephews to keep track of. I was the youngest.

She worked as a corporate secretary until she retired at age 65, and lived in that upstairs apartment for as long as I can remember. She was what my Dad called "A proper lady." She never forgot any of the nieces or nephews birthdays and as they had children and grandchildren of their own, her birthday list became longer and longer.

After my Dad died, she was, pretty much, the only family I had left. I have a bunch of cousins, but for the most part, they are strangers to me. For the last several years of her life, I would call her every other Sunday. We talked about little things; how the weather was in Pennsylvania, what my cousins were up to, and for the last year or two, how my Parkinson's was doing. Her doctor's wife had Parkinson's, so she was familiar with the disease. She and I would often joke that our ages had been switched, I felt like I was in my 90's and she felt like she was still in her 50's. She was a grand lady, that's for sure, and I miss her very much.

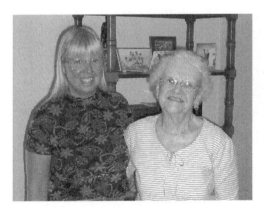

Life Simplified

If there is one thing Parkinson's has taught me, it is that life is simple. I used to have earrings, shoes and handbags that matched all my outfits, now I can't put the earrings in, I only wear Velcro sneakers and my purse is a fanny pack. Simple.

I used to put on eyeliner and mascara, but the Goth look isn't flattering on a 51-year old woman, so now I don't wear any. Simple.

My clothes were home made, designed by me, with intricate buttons and ties and fit perfectly. No more, now its jeans, tank tops and blouses knotted at the waist. Simple.

I used to order steak, rice pilaf and veggies at restaurants, I still order steak, but my Wonderful Husband cuts it for me and I stick to side dishes that can be eaten with fingers. Simple.

I used to wear jewelry, lots of it, but I can't manipulate the clasps now and I don't miss it a bit. The same can be said for styling my hair, it gets combed and that's about it. Simple.

My days start at 4 am and end at 11pm, during those eighteen plus hours, I go through a range of symptoms and I make my life as easy as possible for me.

I have chairs that fit me, not some grand design, my floors are rug free so I don't trip, I have a set of lightweight plastic dishes that I use and my pill bottles are lined up on the counter next to the fridge so I can get to them easily. Simple.

My Wonderful Husband understands when I take a nap at 9 am, while he's just got up and made the bed at eight. Our days are not regimented except for my meds. We generally wing it. Simple.

You should try it.

Yuma Bev's Reality TV Show

Parkinson's requires me to tell my doctors HOW I am doing and I need someone to tell me WHAT I am doing. Sound confusing? It isn't really. Since there are no lab tests to measure our disease, our doctors have to rely on what we tell them is happening to us (and the little bit they observe during our brief visits). I know how I FEEL but don't know how I LOOK, unless I fill my house with mirrors, set up cameras everywhere or get a job in a reality TV show (The Shaky Housewives of PD).

It sounds crazy, but except to comb my hair in the morning, I never SEE myself during the day. I didn't have a clue what I looked like, until I set up a video camera and recorded myself doing my normal things…using a computer, trying to write, watching TV and walking. It was boring stuff, until I watched the recordings.

I never knew my right foot does a weird snake like dance in the air when I try to do anything with my right hand. I had no idea I was walking with my arm flailing outward. I know my arm gets jerky in the evenings, but didn't know the amount it jerks depends on the intensity of what I am watching on TV. If I watch Criminal Minds, my arm jerks like crazy, an old black and white comedy and it moves very little. I had no idea I was sitting there watching TV every night with my mouth hanging open and my head cricked to one side.

It was scary seeing myself, but educational. According to my Wonderful Husband, I don't make these movements all day, just at certain times, and some are worse than others. He says sometimes I sit quite still. It looks painful, but isn't, so at least that's one thing to smile about. The other bonus is all the extra calories I burn.

I don't have these extreme movements all day long, just when my medications are at their peak. YES, these jerky movements are side effects. However, the last one, my mouth hanging open, is caused by the Parkinson's.

I'm Laughing at Parkinson's

I wrote my first song about Parkinson's shortly after I started the Humor blog. I wanted an upbeat tune and fun lyrics so I picked *Tulsa Time* for the melody and these are the lyrics I came up with.

Laughing at Parkinson's

When I was diagnosed
At the age of forty-seven
With this thing they call Parkinson's
I could barely get dressed
I should have been depressed
But I'm laughing at Parkinson's

So I started fighting
And I began by writing
New words to songs just for fun
Then I came out swinging
And I started singing
I'm laughing at Parkinson's

I'm laughing at Parkinson's
I'm laughing at Parkinson's
One day I heard a rumor
You can beat it using humor
So I'm laughing at Parkinson's

I'm zigging and I'm zagging
My right foot is a dragging
My legs feel like they weigh a ton
My hands are a shaking
When I am out picture taking
But I'm laughing at Parkinson's

I ain't no longer clogging
So I started blogging
And funny stories are being spun
When my body wants to wiggle
Then I begin to giggle
'Cuz I'm laughing at Parkinson's

I'm laughing at Parkinson's
I'm laughing at Parkinson's
One day I heard a rumor
You can beat it using humor
So I'm laughing at Parkinson's

I performed it for all my friends at the RV Park where I used to live, the same place I sang Another One Leaves the Park, a few years back. They were used to my absurd song parodies and I wasn't sure what they would think about a song about Parkinson's, but I needn't have been worried. They loved it and gave me a standing ovation. In fact, the music video of this song is me performing it live, that night. It's one of the most viewed videos on my YouTube channel.

Strange Side Effects

I am different than most Young Onset Parkinson's patients and that difference may explain my sense of humor. I went eight years without a diagnosis or any medicines to relieve my symptoms and even as I got worse and the doctors kept saying - "I don't know." I was still optimistic. Just before diagnosis, my symptoms were very similar to Muhammad Ali, I was almost frozen like a statue (Liberty, Venus, Joan Rivers), but I was still alive, whatever I had wasn't fatal, so what was there to be sad about?

Most Parkies take drugs early on; when a tremor is their only symptom and some don't realize they are getting worse, and therefore, don't appreciate how much the medicines are working. Some even say, "I'd have to quit taking them to tell if there is any difference." I know, absolutely, that mine are helping me AND causing some of my problems.

They help my stiffness and shakes, but cause my sleepless nights and two really aggravating things: dyskinesia and dystonia, big words that are hard to spell and even harder to pronounce.

Dyskinesia is a dopamine side effect and is a jerky, dance-like movement of the arms, legs and or head. In other words, I wiggle around like Michael J. Fox. I call it doing the "Parkie Dance" and I can do a good job of timing the movements to music.

Dystonia is muscle contractions and are caused by medicine withdrawal or too much medicine (another oxymoron). I get severe cramps that cause my foot to try to turn itself inside out and tend to happen while crossing a busy street. These have been helped recently by eating bananas and doing stretches, advice I got from Barbara G., a physical therapist who took time to visit the Parkinson's chat room and answer questions we had.

You see, the whole trick with Parkinson's is to figure out how to relieve some symptoms without causing worse ones and it's like standing on someone's shoulders as they ride a bike across a tightrope. It ain't easy! But it can be done!

I was going to write a song parody about dystonia, to the tune of My Sharona, but haven't gotten around to it. Sorry, now you have that song in your head, don't you?

I am lucky, so far, I have not showed any signs of the obsessive /compulsive disorders that plague many who take the medicines. Unless, making people laugh is my side effect. Nope, been doing that all my life!

So, Don't Worry, Be Happy! Now you have this song stuck in your head instead!!

31

Rub a Dub-Dub

Sometimes I forget I have Parkinson's. I did just that one day and the final result is this story. I was feeling kind of stiff and achy (a normal occurrence for me). My Wonderful Husband had gone out jeeping with the neighbors, so I had the whole house to myself.

I was being lazy, watching TV, when a commercial came on showing a nice bubble bath. Wow, I thought, that looks fantastic! I bet a nice hot bath would feel really good. Gee, I haven't taken a bubble bath in years and this new house I live in has a tub in the guest bathroom that has never even been used.

So, I found something I could use as bubble bath and filled the tub. I put on some soothing tunes and climbed in. Ahhhh, it felt sooo good. I could feel myself relaxing and all the stiffness melting away. It was absolutely enjoyable.

That is, until the water cooled off and my skin began to take on that prune look. I tried to get up and out of the tub. Oops. What have I done?

I could not get myself up. There was nothing to grab a hold of to pull myself up. The towel bar was too far away. The sides of the tub were slick fiberglass. There was a small grab bar but it was on my "wrong" side and only about ten-inches above the tub.

There I was, stuck in the tub.

The cell phone was out on the kitchen counter. The neighbors on both sides were out somewhere in the desert with my Wonderful Husband. HELP!

Since panic would only make things worse, and I was now freezing, I ran some more hot water. I started wriggling and twisting around until I was facing the other direction. Finally, after another hour, I managed to get up on my good knee and grabbed the little bar with my good hand. I grabbed the water spigot with the other hand and managed to get myself up enough to climb out of the tub.

By then, I was exhausted, so I took a nap. By the time my Wonderful Husband and the neighbors came home, I was fine and had turned my misadventure into a funny story to be shared over pizza, even joking about the group of handsome Firemen coming to my rescue. That's just me; I find humor anywhere I can.

I did stop by the local firehouse just to check. Nice fellows, but no handsome movie star hunks, so I haven't taken any more baths.

You Can't Fool Grandma

I look healthy and except for the Parkinson's, am healthy. I can sometimes fool younger folks but I can't fool the older ones. If there is one thing I've learned in life, it is never under-estimate senior citizens. They watch over me and know instantly whether I am doing good or bad, especially the women.

I used to live in an RV Park filled with seniors, and if they noticed that I was having trouble, they would come rescue me in a golf cart. Of course, they would never say they were rescuing me; they would come up with a good excuse to give me a ride home.

The ladies were more creative: "Hey I need your advice, can I give you a ride while we talk?" or "Can you show me where Ann lives, she's near you, right?"

The men were more fun. They would say things like: "My wife isn't looking, can I give a ride to the prettiest girl in the park?" or "Let's stir up some gossip, will you ride with me?". These were extremely funny to me, since I knew their wives had sent them to get me, but I played along. I no longer live there and I miss all my friends and the golf cart rides.

Now I live in a new housing community and I walk every morning with George, a neighbor of mine who is 78-years young and his wife, Freida. Some days we walk for forty-five minutes, some days we only do ten, it all depends on how we feel.

34

We watch the sunrise, check out the new construction and see how people have decorated their homes and yards. Sometimes, we even get to see a cactus blooming, but the best part of all is sharing stories and laughing! What a great way to start the day!

While Everyone Sleeps

There is one thing many Parkies have in common, sleep abnormalities. I had Parkinson's for at least eight years before getting diagnosed and never had trouble sleeping; in fact, sleeping was the one thing I could do to relieve my symptoms. Exactly three months after I started taking prescription medicine for my symptoms, I started waking up early, very early, like before Mr. Sunshine even thinks about showing his bright face over the mountains to my east. This lack of sleep should have made me grumpy, but it did not. My humor was intact, maybe more so.

The first morning I awoke early was New Years Day of 2008 and I got a crazy idea. I had a bench in my yard that I put toy bears on (more thrift store goodies), dressed up for the holidays and I had bears dressed in formal wear for New Year's Eve, the night before. It was about 4 am and I knew that none of my neighbors would be stirring at this hour, heck; most had just gone to bed.

So, I started searching for what I needed. I went down to the community hall and found empty beer cans and party favors, and then I raided my own closet, my costume box and some household items. By 5 am, I had all I needed and re-set the bears for the neighbors to wake up to, and what a wake-up it was. Their laughter and hooting woke up my Wonderful Husband about 7 am, poor fellow. By noon, cars from the neighboring communities were driving through, taking pictures.

You see, my bears had a wild night, they were in their underwear, Mr. Bear was hanging upside down with a lampshade on his head and Mrs. Bear was passed out with Mr. Bear's pants on her head. There were empty beer cans all around. Oh, my!!! It was shocking. Especially since the bears owner (me) did not drink, at all. Some people thought that someone else had done it and that I would be upset. Boy, did I have them fooled! Many more holiday "mornings after" followed and neighbors began to look forward to what I would come up with next. I had a blast, while everyone else slept.

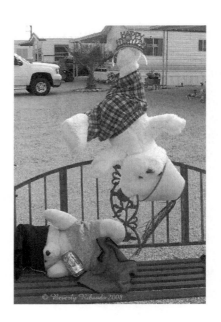

Yuma Bev Makes the News

When my Parkinson's Humor blog was about five weeks old, our local NBC station, KYMA, contacted me about doing a story on me. Christi (and a camera-man) came out to my home and spent an hour or so with me, talking and filming. The interview was divided up between two newscasts later that same day, the 5 pm and 10 pm editions. I still, to this day, don't have any idea how they even found out about my blog, but I am glad they did, because my story brought several new Parkies to our next support group meeting. Here are the transcripts:

KYMA Early News:

Anchor: Well, one woman's fight against Parkinson's disease has taken her into cyberspace and News 11's Christi Rodriguez has her inspiring story.

Christi: Inspiring it is, Bev Ribaudo got diagnosed with Parkinson's disease about four years ago, from that moment, she had no idea that a little bit of humor and the click of a mouse would go such a long way. Ribaudo suffered for years with the symptoms of Parkinson's before any doctor was able to diagnose it. She finally learned she had the disease from a doctor here in Yuma.

One of the side effects from the medication for the disease is a loss of sleep, so one restless night; Ribaudo was online and wandered into a Parkinson's chat room. There she met a fellow Parkie, as she calls them, who inspired her to share her sense of humor with others who were suffering with the disease.

"She said 'Why don't you write a blog?' Well, I had no idea how to write a blog, but she helped me and I got started and I thought, well, it's a good way to show people that just because you have Parkinson's, it doesn't mean it's a death sentence or you should mope around, you can still laugh and enjoy life." says Ribaudo.

Christi: Ribaudo's blog is called Parkinson's Humor and has almost 1300 readers worldwide. Coming up on Nightside, I'll tell you how her blog has reached people on four continents and I'll also have more on Bev's incredible story.

KYMA Nightside News:

Anchor: A Yuma woman diagnosed with Parkinson's disease four years ago isn't letting it get in her way, with a little bit of humor and her computer, she is sharing her story. News 11's Christi Rodriguez introduces us to the woman.

Christi: After her diagnosis, Mrs. Ribaudo set out to find others with her disease as well. She stumbled upon a Parkinson's chat room where she found countless others with the disease, from all over the world. She was able to let the keys do the talking and quickly set her self apart from the rest. Bev quickly earned the reputation for being the chat room clown.

"I would always tell people my little funny jokes and stories on the chat room" says Ribaudo.

A fellow chatter took notice, she suggested to Bev that she should start a blog, and so, Parkinson's Humor was born, but Bev never could have predicted how fast or how far her blog would spread.

"I wrote the first couple stories and I emailed it to, like maybe ten people I know who have Parkinson's, and within a week or two, I

39

looked and it's like, there's people reading my blog from Singapore and Pakistan and Germany. I'm trying to figure out how these people are even finding out about my blog" says Ribaudo.

One of the subjects Ribaudo writes about in her blog is about side effects of medications she is taking and she says "The whole trick is to figure out how to relieve some symptoms without causing worse ones and it's like standing on someone's shoulders as they ride a bike across a tightrope. It ain't easy! But it can be done!" This kind of sunny outlook is perhaps the reason why Bev has almost 1300 readers.

"It seems like all of a sudden, within a month, people all over the world have been reading my little stories from Yuma, Arizona" says Ribaudo, laughing.

Bev doesn't care about numbers as much as she does bringing awareness to the disease, and if she gets a laugh out of it, she'll take that too.

"That's really my goal, to make people see that even though this is a degenerative disease, and there is no cure, it doesn't mean your life is over with. You can still laugh, you can still joke, you can still have a good time, you just have to adapt, and laughter is good medicine for everybody." says Ribaudo.

Well, that is true indeed. If you or someone you know suffers from the disease, there is a local support group right here in Yuma. They meet the first Monday of every month. For more information, you can call the number on the screen.

Anchor: Thank you Christi, I like that positive attitude she has.

Stiff as a Board

The proper term is rigidity, however, just plain stiff is a better description and it is now my main symptom of Parkinson's.

This stiffness can be hard to describe to someone who has never felt it. Muscles normally contract when they are in use, and then relax when they are at rest. In Parkinson's, the muscles of an affected area are always contracted and won't relax. That's why you see us with our hands clenched into a fist sometimes.

When my medicines start to wear off, I can feel my neck stiffen and then the stiffness spreads to my right arm and both legs, making it hard to rise from a seated position. If I tried to come up with a description, I'd say it feels like concrete drying or maybe being starched. Do people use starch anymore? Probably the best way to describe it is like when you are wearing very tight and stiff clothing, like heavy jeans or a thick winter coat; you try to bend your legs or arms and they just won't bend. Anyways, it's a distinct feeling. Kind of like when you have a bad fever, but without the chills and sweating. Things just tighten up. This tightness is very tiring.

Not fun, not at all like getting stiff from booze. Hmmm, wonder if getting drunk would counteract it? I doubt it; I'd probably end up a stiff stiff with a bad hangover.

Stretching is a good way to counteract the tightness. Exercise may be the best medicine for us and it is free.

41

However, you should concentrate on exercises that stretch your muscles instead of contracting them, since the Parkinson's contracts them for you.

When I sleep at night, I try to keep my right hand open wide, either under my pillow or against my leg, depending on which side I am sleeping on. Why? So I don't wake up with a fist I cannot open. I usually have a distinct handprint on my leg from the hand contracting during the night; don't be alarmed, it disappears quickly.

I make one heck of a scarecrow on Halloween!

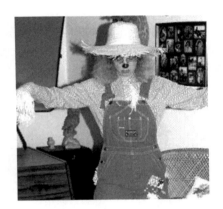

Christmas Cards from the Emergency Room

My parents were older than my friends' parents, older than their grandparents in some cases, and I only remember them with gray hair, probably caused by five accident prone kids, of which I was the youngest.

We didn't have typical childhood accidents, we were creative, we did things like fall off two story buildings and the back of motorcycles, we roller-skated carrying bags of glass bottles and fell down (thereby not only breaking bones but also getting cut badly) and we came home with our pockets full of poisonous snakes, scorpions, etc., you name it and one of us got bit or stung by it.

We got hit by cars and burned by fires and we rode our bicycles ... into telephone pole guy wires, closed gates, off the roof of the house and the best one ... performed by yours truly ... headfirst into the side of a UPS truck. That little stunt earned me my first flight in a helicopter, but I was out cold and missed the whole ride. I also got to meet a former U.S. President due to that trick, but that's another story.

Mom, however, always planned ahead, and each time we moved to a new base (Dad was in the Air Force), she would bake a bunch of goodies and go introduce herself to the emergency room staff of the hospital, since she knew she'd be a regular. Within months, they knew her by name and would cringe when she came through the door dragging one of us along.

We were such memorable patients that Mom got Christmas cards from them for years after! Not the normal, "I hope all is well" Christmas cards, these were "Are the kids still alive?" and "I am glad you got transferred to another base" kinds of cards!

Amazingly, we all survived childhood.

Shake, Shake, Shake

I remember seeing a group of men with musical instruments at a bluegrass festival in the early 90's. This one man's hands were shaking terribly, so badly, I was afraid he wouldn't be able to pick up his squeeze-box (a small accordion type instrument) that sat next to his chair. I was right. The fellow next to him picked it up and placed the strap around his neck. The music started and this man carefully and with much difficulty placed his hands on it and began to play. As soon as he grasped the squeeze box, the shaking stopped and he played flawlessly. It was incredible to watch and the group got a standing ovation when they were done, but as soon as he quit playing, the horrid shakes were back and the man next to him, helped him put the instrument away.

I knew the gentleman had Parkinson's, I'd seen shaking hands before. I went up to him and praised his playing. He told me he was only 86 and had been playing since he was a child. Neither of us mentioned the shaking hands.

Tremors are the most common and easily recognized symptom of Parkinson's. Almost all of us Parkies have them at some time or other. They come in three flavors, resting, action and internal. I've had them all. The gentleman above had the most common type, resting. His hands only shook when he wasn't using them, when they were at rest.

I started with the action type, my right hand was fine, until I tried to use it and then it would shake uncontrollably. This made it very difficult to write, drink and eat. I was forever picking up food off the floor and spilling my drink. I started using my left hand and soon became so proficient that people thought I was a true lefty. I never mastered writing left handed, so I gave up writing and my Wonderful Husband took over the writing jobs; checks, grocery lists and even Christmas cards (I can't say I miss that last one).

The only time I have the resting type tremors are when I am tired (and then it is slight) or if I am very upset, then my whole right arm shakes uncontrollably, so I try to avoid arguments and traffic accidents.

I have occasionally had internal tremors. The best way I can describe them is it feels like parts of me are shivering. This can be absurd when the thermometer reads 112 degrees outside.

Tremors are not always a bad thing. I do one heck of a job making scrambled eggs and milk shakes. If I could time my tremors to music, I bet I'd be an excellent tambourine player and if James Bond happens to stop by, I can make him a martini, shaken not stirred.

How Do I Explain Parkinson's to a Cat?

Cat is a beautiful young lady from West Virginia, U.S.A., who contacted me through Twitter and asked if I could answer some questions she had about Parkinson's. I said yes and the emails began, but there was just one problem, Cat is blind, she has been since birth, so describing Parkinson's became a challenge.

Cat and I have some things in common: We both have a wicked sense of humor, she wants a t-shirt that says "Don't stare at me, I can't stare back" and I want one that says "What's shaking? Besides me?" We both like Michael J. Fox and would like to meet him someday. She refers to him as Mr. Fox, because her parents taught her manners and I refer to him as Michael J., because I am older than him.

We have our differences as well: She is shy and self-conscious about her looks and I am definitely not shy and don't give a hoot what people think about me, but that comes with age. I am old enough to be her mother.

Cat "reads" what's on her computer by using software that vocalizes what is on the screen, kind of like books on tape. She read some of my early blog stories and her question was about tremors: were they caused by the Parkinson's or the medicines we take and what is the difference between tremors and dyskinesia? (There's that really big word, again)

The first part of the question was easy; the Parkinson's

causes tremors. Describing the difference was going to be harder. This is what I came up with:

Tremors are like when your hands shake because you are nervous or scared and can be similar to shivering or having the chills when you get a fever. Sitting on them or if someone else holds them still can stop shaking hands or fingers.

Dyskinesia or The Wiggles, as I call them, are caused by the medicines we take to stop the tremors and are sort of like trying to hold on to a squirming child that does NOT want to be held. You can't stop it! If my Wonderful Husband grabs my moving hand and holds it still, the movement goes to my arm and if he holds both my arm and hand still, the movement goes to my upper body. Your body is going to move, usually in a rhythmic fashion, almost like rocking, so I just go with it. Fortunately, it doesn't last long, at least not for me.

I thought it was a pretty good explanation.

You can find both of us on Twitter, I am @YumaBev and Cat is @gilman_gal. Give us a Tweet, but be sure to mention this story, so we know how you found us.

By the way, if any of you know Mr. Michael J. Fox personally, please tell him we said Hello.

Cat says that she thinks she prefers blindness to Parkinson's, I don't agree, but that's okay. We can still be friends.

Humor Also Runs in the Family

Not only did my Dad have Parkinson's too, but, he could be just as wacky as I am. I have a photo of my Dad, dressed as a woman, jumping out of a giant present at an office Christmas party. I was about ten at the time and Mom and I thought it was hilarious. He had a very dry sense of humor and loved to embarrass and tease me. He would introduce me as his wife...or say I was his son George, both of which would elicit a piercing "Daaaadddd" from me, which would just make him laugh.

 When I complained about being called "Beverly Hillbillies" by the kids in school, my Dad would say "I wanted to name you Chrysanthemum, but I couldn't spell it and your Mom didn't like Marigold Petunia, so I wouldn't complain about Beverly."

Years later, when I married my Wonderful Husband and became step-mom to two young adults who were almost my age, my Dad quickly figured out that if he would marry my step-daughter, then I would become his mother-in-law and he could be his own grandfather!

Dad proposed, my step-daughter said NO!

Parts, Parts and More Parts

What parts of your body might be affected by Parkinson's? Any part of your body you can voluntarily move MIGHT be affected, as well as some parts of your body that move on their own. That doesn't mean they WILL be affected. It all depends on your squirrel in your dashboard.

An online Parkie friend sums it up very well. She says that we Parkies are all in the same boat, we are just on different lakes. Some folks still have a working boat motor, some are using two oars, some just have one paddle and others are really "up the creek without a paddle." It all depends on your particular squirrel, as well as the time of day and how long you have had Parkinson's.

My day usually starts with a working motor and then settles somewhere between two oars and a paddle. I have been up the creek without a paddle, but it could be worse, I could be in the ocean during a hurricane!

So, what are some of the weird parts that can be affected?

How about eyelids? Yup, we tend to blink less and that can cause vision problems due to dryness.

How about curling toes? Sometimes they really curl under or up, sometimes it just feels like they have and they are perfectly straight.

How about your bladder? Yes, I said bladder. You know

the commercial for men with prostate problems, talking about difficulty starting the stream? It can happen with Parkinson's.

I know this because it happens to me. I feel like I really need to "go", but can't get it started. So, I use a trick I learned from the Alzheimer's people. I hung pictures of waterfalls all over my bathroom walls. It works every time. Why? A different part of your brain reacts to photos. For the same reason, some Parkies who have difficulty starting to walk will do fine if they hear music or hum a marching band type song. It all has to do with rerouting the garbled communications.

Every day is different with Parkinson's, but by the end of the day, I can always find something to laugh about. I hope you can, too, even if you are NOT a Parkie.

My Pikes Peak Adventure

We had been to Colorado Springs, Colorado several times during the years we lived and travelled in an RV, but we never went to the top of Pikes Peak, so it remained on my Bucket List until the fall of 2011. I was feeling good, so we took an impromptu vacation and drove to Colorado. When it came to summiting Pikes Peak, we had two choices: drive up in our car, nineteen miles one way with 53 hairpin turns and no guardrails or we could sit back and take a narrated tour on the Cog Railway. We elected for the train so we could both enjoy the scenery. The narration was great.

I did not ask my doctor whether the 14,110 ft altitude would affect my Parkinson's; I never gave it a thought. I knew it would be cold up there, thirty degrees colder than where you boarded the train, so I packed two jackets each for my Wonderful Husband and me. The ride to the top took approximately one and a half hours and the scenery was absolutely beautiful, the aspens were bright yellow, the sky brilliant blue with white puffy clouds. We saw deer, marmots, waterfalls, alpine lakes and my favorite tree, the blue spruce.

I felt fine, until we almost reached the top. I had chosen the departure time to be the warmest part of the day, since cold aggravates my Parkinson's symptoms and to be in the "best" part of a medicine cycle. All of a sudden, my left foot began to cramp and my neck stiffened. I checked my pill container and yes, I HAD taken my pills right on time. What was going on? I should be as fluid as

I get during a dosing period, but instead it was as if I hadn't taken any medicine at all. By the time we reached the summit, ten minutes later, I was very rigid and both feet were cramping. I felt like a 100-year old lady.

I got off the train and slowly made my way into the gift shop and headed straight for the bathroom, along with every other woman on the train. It took me forever to get there, shuffling along and of course, there was a long line, so I just took my place. Soon, someone was tapping me on my shoulder, it was an employee, and she led me out of line and to a handicapped stall and said, "I think this will be better for you." I was thankful and a bit embarrassed. I think some of the passengers probably thought I was faking, but I wasn't. I could barely move.

After using the facilities, I managed to walk around a bit and snap some pictures, I ate a high altitude doughnut (yummy) and posed for a picture or two and then it was time (thankfully) to get back on the train for the ride down. Once we got below the 10,000 ft point, I felt everything relaxing and the cramping disappeared. I felt better by the time we reached the bottom, but I was exhausted (your entire body contracting is very tiring). We stopped and picked up some dinner to go and went back to the hotel and went to bed early.

Would I do it all over again? Absolutely! The scenery was spectacular. Wouldn't you be willing to "suffer" a bit to see something so beautiful?

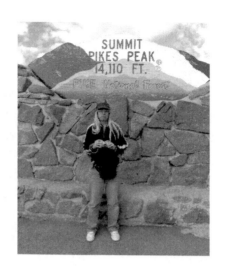

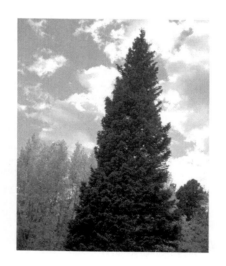

Wild and Crazy Moomer

My humor came from my Dad, but I got my craziness from my Mom. Moomer (that's what everyone called her) was the most outrageous person I ever knew. She got scolded as a teen for jazzing up the hymns on the church organ and caused a scandal by showing up at the town pool in a homemade bikini. It was no big deal to her, but in 1936, it was shocking to everyone else!

She was ahead of her time, she listened to pop and rock radio and won tickets to a Rolling Stones concert in 1981. She went to the concert and had a blast, she was only 62! While everyone else was getting stoned, she was drinking coke spiked with Geritol.

She bought me wigs, crocheted me bikinis, made me wild outfits and called the school officials "old fuddy-duddies" when I did something inappropriate at school. She made two sets of clothes for me, wild ones and plain ones and told people I was a twin. One day, she couldn't pick me up at school, so she sent our neighbor (a Highway Patrolman) to get me. He showed up, in his uniform, with lights flashing and took me out in handcuffs and put me in the back of the cruiser. The two of them laughed about it for hours and I was "'totally cool" the next day at school!

She might have been older, but she was the coolest Mom around. She loved to laugh; dance and make silly faces and all my friends wished their Moms were like mine.

She is the reason I feel comfortable singing my wacky song parodies, dressing up in silly costumes and writing these stories! I wish she were here to read them.

I miss you, Moomer.

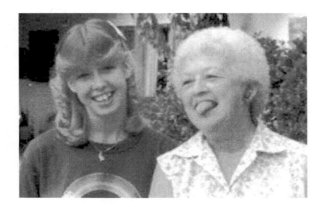

All the Skinny on This Parkie

I am fairly healthy, except for Parkinson's, but I still spend a lot of time in doctors' offices. The medicines I take for Parkinson's can cause melanoma, so I see a lady dermatologist twice a year for a complete skin check. I've had two cancers cut off my nose already. She treats my Rosacea, as well (that's why my face looks red all the time).

Dr. L. comes in, looks me over and scolds me because my arms and legs are darkly tanned. I tell her that I can't help it. I tan really fast. She looks puzzled and says "But you are blonde. Are you a natural blonde? Of course you are, even your eyelashes are blonde. How long does it take for you to see a difference in color?"

Ten minutes, I answer.

"In ten minutes? You see a difference? That doesn't make sense, you have fair skin, and you shouldn't tan at all." I just shrug my shoulders. Dr. L. is almost as white as the paper gown I am wearing.

The hair on my body is short, baby fine and blonde and I have so little of it that I don't have to shave my legs! Yippee! This amazes Dr. L.: she just can't believe it. She says I am the least hairy adult she has ever seen and asks if I have always been like that. No, I answer, I used to have thick black hair all over me. She looks puzzled again, and then laughs. I'm not sure she understands my weird sense of humor.

57

I have always been different, my fingernails are see-through and bend and nail polish will not stick to them. My baby toenail is so tiny that I can barely cut it. My hair and parts of my face are very oily and the rest of my skin is very dry.

What can I say? I am an anomaly, I shouldn't tan, but I do. I shouldn't have Parkinson's either, but I do. I shouldn't be a Happy Parkie, but I am.

Good Things about Having Parkinson's

I asked several of my fellow Parkies to come up with good things about having Parkinson's, turns out they have a sense of humor, too. Here are some of their replies and a few of my own:

My husband now dusts the knick-knacks in the china cabinet because I was breaking too many of them.

I don't even notice when the batteries die in my electric toothbrush, because I shake so much.

I get new dishes every few months because I break so many of them.

I got all new shirts with snaps instead of buttons.

No one thinks twice when I drink wine out of a Sippy cup.

I get a handicapped-parking permit.

Elastic waist pants with over-sized t-shirts.

They send me to watch football with the guys on Thanksgiving instead of helping in the kitchen.

I have a great excuse to not shave my legs anymore.

When I fall down, while I am lying on the floor, I check for dust bunnies under the furniture.

Someone else checks the eggs at the grocery store and picks the oranges off the fancy pyramid stacker, ever since "the incident."

I don't need a blender to make a margarita; I shake enough on my own.

I never get asked to pour the wine or champagne or even the iced tea at dinner.

No one will open the can of beer or cola I just got from the refrigerator.

I don't get asked to change diapers or feed babies.

I buy Velcro shoes.

I can Shake-N-Bake like no body else.

My young kids want to learn how Mommy does "The Shake" dance.

Living in an RV

For sixteen years (1991 - 2006), my Wonderful Husband and I lived in an RV (recreational vehicle) and traveled all over the U.S.A. and most of Canada. I would still be doing it, if I did not have Parkinson's. Many people have expressed curiosity about RVs, mostly from other countries, but several Americans as well. So, here is the story.

We bought our first RV in 1991, a 21-foot long motor home (Motor home means that it has its own engine and you drive it like a car) and took off on a three week trip. There wasn't much room in it, you had to make a bed out of the sofa every night and you couldn't pass each other in the hallway, but after two weeks, we didn't want to go home, ever, so, we traded it for a 34 foot motor home and kept on traveling.

This RV was small inside as well, but it had a full size bed in it (you had about six-inches on either side to walk around) and a sofa and dinette, so we thought we were in heaven.

Several years later, we got rid of the motor home and from then on, we had a variety of RVs that you towed behind or placed in the bed of a truck. Sometimes, we would buy a very small one to take a specific trip and then sell it after we were done, it all depended on where we were going, but we lived in an RV of some kind or another year round.

The last RV we owned was the biggest and we towed it behind a big pick up truck; however, it was still only about 200-square feet of living space. For most RVers in America, this would be called a weekender, just big enough for two or three days, but we lived in it for seven years! I did 99% of the driving and could back it into the tightest spaces.

It was still very small inside, and to give you some perspective, a doorway inside an RV is about twenty-inches wide and one inside my house is thirty. Ten-inches make a huge difference.

The space for walking was quite narrow in the bedroom and bathroom and as my Parkinson's symptoms progressed, it became increasingly difficult for me to manage without constantly bumping into things. The entry steps to get in the camper were tricky as well and I didn't feel comfortable towing the RV anymore, so we gave up that life and started a new one. Adapt, adapt, adapt.

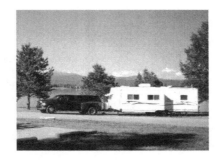

A Funny Thing Happened on My Way Back From...

We went to Laughlin, Nevada, to watch the National Karaoke Finals in September and after the elimination rounds were over each evening, they had karaoke in the casino's lounge. I know it sounds funny, but the contestants (I was NOT one of them) just couldn't wait to get into party mode after spending hours being in competition mode and they were fun to watch.

I wanted to sing one of my funny song parodies, but by 10 pm, I was worn out. What happened to that Disco Queen that used to start partying at 10 pm? Oh, yeah, right, I forgot, duh, I have Parkinson's. I'm absolutely sure it has nothing to do with being 51-years old!

The Emcee would play a "real" song every once in awhile and she played *Thriller*, by Michael Jackson. I had gone to the ladies room and on my way back, I took a short cut across the dance floor, which was almost empty.

All of a sudden, people started clapping and cheering. I looked around and they were cheering at me.

I didn't know it, but while I was in the ladies room, they had called an impromptu dance contest and the people thought I was dancing. They were shouting "She's doing the Mummy" and "She looks like Lurch from the Addams Family."

63

I wasn't dancing at all, I was just walking (stiffly) back to my chair, but being me, I got into the spirit of things and I tried to time my steps to the music (not easy). Everyone was clapping and I was pronounced the winner!!!

I stayed in character and stiffly climbed up on stage to take a bow and then "Lurched" my way back to my seat.

It's a good thing they didn't ask me to Moonwalk!

A Halloween Party in Cyberspace

I spent a lot of time visiting with other Parkies in a Parkinson's chat room and there was a really good reason. The people on there like to have fun. They had a party for Halloween night, an online party, anyone with a computer and Internet could attend and you didn't even have to leave home. The host of the party, Steve, played YouTube clips of the *Monster Mash* and *Teen Wolf* with Michael J. Fox. We told silly jokes and laughed at our real or Photoshop created costumes and for a little while, we were able to forget Parkinson's and just have fun.

As a surprise for this party, I wrote a song about a Halloween party and I picked out costumes for a whole bunch of my online friends. Then, using their Facebook profile photos and Photoshop, I "put" them in the costumes and made a music video of my song and Steve played it at the party. We had some great laughs and I think they all enjoyed it. They all seemed tickled by the costumes I chose for each. What did I create for myself? I did a sexy Mae West type gown with a feather boa. What? You were expecting a clown?

Holiday Advice for Friends and Family

With some big holidays approaching, I want to share some advice from a person living with Parkinson's to all my friends and family who don't know exactly what I go through each day. Please invite me to join you for whatever you have planned. Don't assume that I won't feel well enough to attend, but please try to understand why I may say no.

I have difficulty with fine motor skills, so please stop and think before you ask me to serve liquids or help put away those crystal wine glasses, there is nothing fun about breaking glass or spilled gravy. I have trouble-cutting meat-into bite size pieces and maneuvering peas from the plate to my mouth, so I do much better with finger foods and stuff that won't fall off the fork when my hands won't cooperate. I feel uncomfortable eating around strangers, they tend to stare, and I know they can't help it, I find myself staring at people, too.

I really should take my "dopamine" medicine on an empty stomach. It works better that way. Pretty much my entire daily routine is dictated by taking my medicines. I'm on a three times a day schedule.

A typical day consists of waking at 5 am; I take medications at 6 am, 2 pm, and 10 pm, so I try to eat at 8:30 am, 12:30 pm and 6 pm. I usually go to bed around 11 pm.

As you can see, eating a huge meal at 2 pm will just throw my day out of whack, but sometimes I do it anyway.

I can go from "on" (which is when my meds are working their best and I feel my best) to "off" (which means they aren't) in ten minutes or less, this explains why I walk into the restaurant just fine, but move slowly going out.

Stress and excitement aggravate my symptoms. Even good stuff, like weddings or other emotional parties can adversely affect me. An argument or shouting will have me shaking from head to toe.

This is why I usually spend the holidays with just my Wonderful Husband. We have a simple meal and a very calm day. It's not that I don't enjoy company; it's just that I do better in more casual situations with smaller groups of people.

Happy Holidays

The Thanksgiving Song

It was early on Wednesday, the day before Thanksgiving and I was chatting online. My friends, mostly Moms, were discussing past holidays. They were lamenting the fact that when their grown-up children come to visit for the Holidays, how little they actually get to see them. "Last year, all my son did was visit his friends," said one. "My daughter showed up with a new boyfriend and spent the whole visit taking him sightseeing," said another. "Yeah," said another, "The only time I see any of them is when they sit down for the turkey dinner and then they shovel it in as fast as they can and disappear."

I sat there, mostly listening, since I don't have any children of my own, but my mind was taking it all in, and the creative side of me was already working. As I listened to their complaints, all valid, a song began to write itself and I knew just the melody to borrow, *Except for Monday* by Lorrie Morgan. I excused myself, signed off, and looked to see if I had a karaoke version of the song and within an hour or two, The Thanksgiving Song was written, recorded and the music video produced. I uploaded it to YouTube and emailed the link to every Mom on my list.

The words must have struck a chord, because it became my most watched video, with over 1,000 views before the Thanksgiving weekend was over. In fact, it's still my most viewed video.

Here are the lyrics.

I was surprised
When you said you were coming
For Thanksgiving
And gonna stay all week

I was so happy
We'd spend time together
Just my daughter and me
All by ourselves

Except on Saturday
You showed up with a boyfriend
Sunday you watched football with him
Monday you took him shopping for a phone
Tuesday and Wednesday you played golf
Thursday you ate and then you took off
And it's Friday now and I'm back to being alone

Don't get me wrong
I really love my family
But I was tired
Of feeling used

It didn't take me long
To make a reservation
So next Thanksgiving
I'll be on a cruise

So, on Saturday
You spend time with your boyfriend
Sunday you watch football with him
Monday take him shopping for new shoes
Tuesday and Wednesday go play golf
Thursday cook the turkey yourself
'Cuz next Thanksgiving
I'll be on a cruise

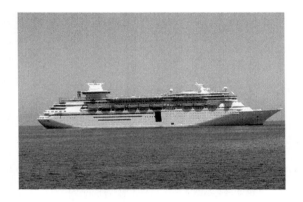

Thanksgiving: What am I Thankful for?

It's 4 am on Thanksgiving morning and I am wide-awake. It's dark outside and very quiet, I don't hear coyotes and even our neighborhood owls aren't hooting. Everyone seems to be sleeping, except me, but I am not complaining. As I sit here in the darkness, I am thinking, not about funny stories or new song parodies, but what all I am thankful for, and the list is long.

My Wonderful Husband: He wakes up alone every morning and hates it, but never complains. He makes sure I get a good meal every day and is a great cook. He goes to karaoke with me, even though being in a noisy bar type atmosphere is the last thing he wants to do, because that's what he did for a living. I don't know how I got so lucky, but I'm glad I did and I love him very much. Thanks for being my best friend.

My Good Neighbors: George & Freida walk with me most mornings, Phil & Ruth and Jim & Carole live on either side of me and are always smiling, Willie & Sharon invite me to all their social functions and all the others who wave and say hello when I stagger past. Thanks for being my friends and making this a nice neighborhood.

My Parkie Friends: They live in Canada, all over the U.S.A., Australia, Europe and the rest of the world. We talk online and I can always count on them to "know" what I am feeling. Plus, they will even listen to my latest song parodies and sometimes even request them. Thanks for being there.

71

My other friends: I am so lucky to have met so many nice people over the years and most keep in touch. If I run into any of them, I can be guaranteed a big hug. I love hugs, the whole world could use more hugs. Thanks for all the hugs.

My Facebook friends who make me smile, my Twitter friends who cheer me up 140 characters at a time, the people at karaoke who laugh at my songs and don't throw tomatoes at me. Thanks!

I am thankful that I just have Parkinson's and not something more serious, that my doctors really seem to care about me, that I haven't lost my sense of humor, that my stepdaughter and grandson are good people, and that I live in America.

I am thankful that I live in Yuma, Arizona where the sun is always shining and it never snows and occasionally, because I am always up early, I get treated to beautiful sunrises like the one I just saw. Life is definitely good.

What are you thankful for?

Yesterday I headed for the store
Needed to get just a few things
But I couldn't remember what I went for
So I sat in the car wondering

Wondering why, I can't remember
If it's May or December
Did I feed the cat
Did I take my nap
Walking all winter wondering

Christmas Eve in Yuma

Since I live in the desert and close to Mexico, people tend to do Christmas a little differently around here. Tamales are a favorite Christmas food and an agave flower spike makes an interesting Christmas tree. Agaves are a cactus that gets a huge flower spike. The dead spikes are treasured as decorations.

They are quite large, sometimes twenty-feet high, and the plant expends so much energy producing the bloom, that the plant dies. It is common to see lights strung on cactus and palm trees and even ornaments hanging on them. Agave spikes make lightweight and interesting Christmas trees.

Santa comes to Yuma in a four-wheel drive vehicle; he leaves Rudolph and the other reindeer up by the Grand Canyon where it's cooler. There are no chimneys, no fireplaces either, it's just too warm, so I'm not sure how he gets in to leave the presents under the agave tree, but if you are good, he figures it out somehow.

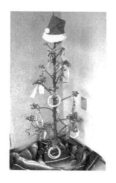

The Twelve Days of Christmas, Parkie Style

On the morning of Christmas, Santa gave to me

Twelve pills to take

Eleven aches and pains

Ten twitching fingers

Nine dropped cookies

Eight shirts I can't button

Seven trips to the bathroom

Six hours of sleep

Five cramping toes

Four hours of wiggles

Three stumbles and falls

Two cold feet

And I'm stiffer than the frozen snowman.

The Seven Dwarfs Come for Christmas

It was a big surprise when we woke up on Christmas morning and found some of the Seven Dwarfs and a few of their cousins had taken up residence. They were as follows: Grumpy, Dopey, Sleepy and Sneezy and they brought along: Coughy, Achy and Sniffley. Yup, you guessed it; my Wonderful Husband woke up with a bad Cold and by the time the day was over, I had it too. We like to do EVERYTHING together.

Colds do not agree with Wonderful Husbands or Parkies. We do not find anything humorous about them. Colds make all Husbands miserable and tend to aggravate the symptoms of people with Parkinson's, since the virus stresses our immune systems. I don't know how a Husband with Parkinson's would be with a Cold, but I don't want to find out.

Later in the morning, another Dwarf showed up at the door. His name was Fevery and we did our best to keep him out, but he got in anyway. We both really hate that one.

Parkinson's medicines come with a huge list of "Do not take with blah, blah, blah" so finding a cold medicine for a Parkie ain't easy. I tend to use my Mom's tried and true remedy, rub Vicks VapoRub on my chest, put on an old t-shirt and go to bed.

Dats juss wha dis Pawkie is gone do. Translation: That's just what this Parkie is going to do; it's hard to talk proper when you have a cold.

Funny thing about all of this, both of our noses are now just as red as Rudolph's!

If you see Snow White, please tell her to come get her Dwarfs.

Dinner with the Neighbors on Christmas Day

In everyone's life there are certain dates on a calendar that make you smile because they remind you of happy events and there are dates that make you sad because they remind you of very bad events. I have many happy dates and only three bad ones. The worst of my bad dates is December 24th and it can't be ignored because it's the day before Christmas. It doesn't matter what happened on this date, it's just the prologue of this story.

Our Christmas tree is about ten-inches high and was made by a dear friend many years ago when we lived in an RV. She died soon after and we put it out each year as a tribute to her. It is the only sign of Christmas in our home and there will be no presents under it. We buy each other gifts whenever we feel like it but never for Christmas and we never put cookies out for Santa.

My Wonderful Husband has similar feelings at Christmas and that's why we don't decorate or buy each other presents. We usually have a big plate of pasta and stay by ourselves.

For the last two years, our very nice neighbors (Phil & Ruth) have invited us for Christmas dinner and we've said no. They invited us again this year and we said yes.

It was just a small gathering, nine, Phil & Ruth, Shirley & Jerry (Ruth's sister & brother-in-law), George & Freida (my walking partners), Erv (another neighbor) and us. It was a planned potluck and each brought their specialty.

We had ham, scalloped potatoes, corn pudding, deviled eggs, Hawaiian sweet potatoes, and three kinds of dessert and a nice bottle of blackberry wine.

We only had one mishap; a glass of wine got knocked over as we finished saying grace. I guess we should have included not spilling anything in our blessing and I was thankful that it wasn't me who did the knocking over. In fact, I didn't drop or spill anything and no one complained when I ate most of my meal with my fingers, since I was having trouble with a fork.

It was a feast and after dinner, we sat around and talked and laughed about all kinds of things until we had room for dessert. Shirley told us about her neighbor who cooked really strange things and always wanted her to try them, Erv told us about growing up on a farm and I even sang a little bit of one of my funny songs. All in all, it was a very enjoyable day, and I thank Phil and Ruth for inviting us.

Add in special thanks, to them, for sending home some leftovers with me, I gobbled them up the next day while my Wonderful Husband stayed in bed with a bad cold.

My Wonderful Husband was much better by the following day and it looks like I didn't catch the cold after all. He says I did a great job as caregiver.

New Year's Eve 2011

My final day of 2011 started when I woke up at 2:30 am, so I went online and watched it turn 2012 in Samoa while I chatted with Kevin in Australia, Cat in West Virginia and Samantha in England. After about an hour, I got sleepy and went back to bed and zonked out. I didn't wake up until 8:15 am, so I missed my first batch of pills for the day by over two hours and for the first time in years; I missed getting to see the sunrise.

My Wonderful Husband took me out to lunch at my favorite restaurant, Famous Dave's BBQ and we had the best meal and then Mimi, the manager, stopped by to say hello and wish us a Happy New Year. Mimi is the greatest.

On the way home, my Wonderful Husband said, "Why don't we have a party tonight and invite the neighbors over?" This surprised me because we both always worked on New Year's Eve, so a party was usually the last thing either one of us wanted to do. I said sure, but it's kind of last minute, they probably all have plans. He gave them a call and all said yes, they'd love to come for a party.

We had pizza and beer and wine and it looked like a frat party when it started, then we all got full and just sat around talking.

Next thing we knew, Dick Clark came on TV and the ball started to drop. We had eaten all the pizza, polished off a bottle of wine and more than a few beers and stayed awake until it was midnight in New York.

We hugged each other and said Happy New Year and clicked our glasses. Then we realized that we were all tired, so our guests headed off toward their various homes.

On his way out, a new neighbor said to me "I think you might have had a little too much tonight" and winked. He thought that my staggering walk was because I was drunk! I just winked back and said, "You might be right!" He doesn't know about the Parkinson's yet and he'll be surprised, if he reads this story, to find out all I drank all night was plain old water!

January 1, 2012

The first day of 2012, started early, as usual. I was receiving lots of emails from Parkies, asking advice about how they could better take care of themselves and since New Year's Day was a great time for resolutions, I made some of my own. First, I would walk everyday, even if I had to walk alone. Second, I would try to sneak useful information into my stories. Keep the stories funny, but educate as well. It would be a challenge, but I felt like it was the right thing to do. So, the first thing I did was write a song called Learning the Parkie Lingo, and then I wrote a story to go with it.

Learning the Parkie Lingo

It won't be easy and the words are hard to pronounce, but you will be a better Parkinson's patient if you learn the medical lingo, so here is a primer. I will try my best to make it fun.

ON - when the medicine IS working and your symptoms are better

OFF - when the medicine is NOT working or has worn off and your symptoms come back

TREMORS - those shaking body parts

RIGIDITY - when you feel like you are in a body cast

DYSTONIA - (dis TOE nee uh) - those severe cramps you get

BRADYKINESIA - (BRADY ki NEE zee uh) - when you move like you are in slow motion

DYSKINESIA - (dis ki NEE zee uh) - those rhythmic movements (like Michael J. Fox) that are a side effect of the dopamine meds

POSTURAL INSTABILITY - when you are stooped over or can't maintain your balance (help, I've fallen and I can't get up)

MASKING - when your face no longer shows emotion (Poker face)

Don't worry about not pronouncing them correctly; just do the best you can. I wrote a song about them, like the song from Mary Poppins: Supercalifragilisticexpialidocious. Once we sang along with her, everyone could pronounce it!

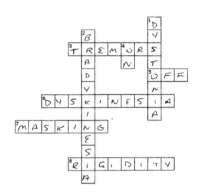

PS This blog story and the song I wrote to go with it became one of the top three most popular and inspired me to write more "educational" type stories.

Charting a Parkie

Most of us with Parkinson's make the same mistake when we go to see our neurologist. We have a conversation like this:

Doctor: How are you doing?

Patient: Fine

Doctor: (to himself, then why are you here?)

Sounds like the start of a joke, doesn't it? It does, but it's not funny.

I used to have conversations like this with my neurologist until I realized that I have to know EXACTLY what is going on with my body so that I can report properly.

About a week before my last appointment, I made a symptom chart and marked on it every hour or so as to what exactly was going on with me. To make it simple, I made columns that depicted my various problems (rigidity, slowness, walking, balance, dexterity, etc.) and chose a number between one and ten to depict how I felt. I also noted when I woke up, took meds, ate, napped, and other general feelings.

I made it using Works, which is the database software on my old PC, but you can use anything. There's probably an app for your phone. I would have written it on a piece of paper, but my writing is worse than any doctor's.

After a few days, I noticed some unusual things:

I would get a headache when my medicine started wearing OFF, then a stiff neck. These both disappeared when I was ON.

I was wearing OFF after about four hours but taking doses six hours apart and it was taking about ninety minutes after a pill to feel ON again, so I was OFF about seven hours a day.

When I was OFF, my nose would be all clogged up but I could breathe just fine when I was ON.

I always felt better right after sleeping or eating a chocolate chip cookie. I thought about just eating cookies, but then I'd get fat and my Wonderful Husband would leave me for a skinny Parkie.

I might not have ever noticed these things had I not taken the time to chart exactly how I felt during the day.

I reported all of this (well, I left out the cookie part) to my neurologist (who was very impressed) and we, yes we, decided to lower the strength of the medicine I was taking and increase the number of pills I take. I went from taking three 150's a day (six hours apart) to taking five 100's a day (four hours apart) and I increased my ON time to almost the whole day and I am only taking 50mg more dopamine type medicine.

Consider charting yourself before your next neurology visit and pay real close attention to how you feel after eating a chocolate chip cookie (maybe I have found a

90

cure).

Keep in mind that what works for me may not work for you and always discuss medicine changes with your doctor.

PS The folks at the Michael J. Fox Foundation loved this story so much, they asked permission to share it on their website, and made me a guest blogger. I said yes, of course.

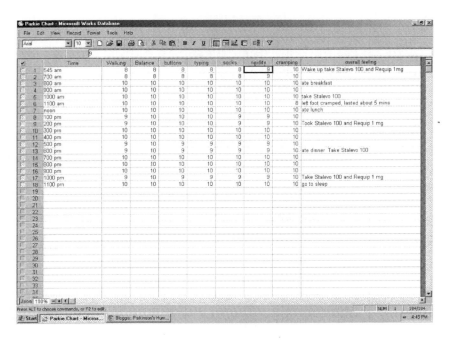

My "after" chart

What If Elvis Had Been a Parkie?

Today, January 8th, 2012 is Elvis' birthday and, as far as I know, he did NOT have Parkinson's. Yesterday, my friend Mickie had an Elvis party in the chat room and last night at my neighbor George's birthday party we were talking about Elvis. So, I woke up this morning and wondered what his songs would have been like if he had Parkinson's and I came up with some humorous results. See for yourself.

ALL SHOOK UP - original lyrics

A well I bless my soul, what's wrong with me? I'm itching like a man on a fuzzy tree

My friends say I'm actin wild as a bug, I'm in love, I'm all shook up. Mm mm oh, oh, yeah, yeah!

My hands are shaky and my knees are weak, I can't seem to stand on my own two feet

Who do you thank when you have such luck? I'm in love, I'm all shook up. Mm mm oh, oh, yeah, yeah!

ALL SHOOK UP - Parkie version

Oh my goodness, What's wrong with me? My hands are shaking like leaves on a tree

My friends say I'm walking like I'm a drunk, I'm a Parkie, I'm all shook up, Mm mm oh oh yeah yeah

My legs are wobbly and my voice is weak, I can't seem to coordinate my two feet

What do you think is causing all this junk? I'm a Parkie, I'm all shook up, Mm mm oh oh yeah yeah

ARE YOU LONESOME TONIGHT - original lyrics

Are you lonesome tonight? Do you miss me tonight? Are you sorry we drifted apart?

Does your memory stray to a brighter sunny day? When I kissed you and called you sweetheart?

ARE YOU TREMBLING TONIGHT - Parkie version

Am I trembling tonight? Does it give you a fright? Are you sorry that you married me?

Do my wiggling arms, cause you much harm, when I kiss you and miss you completely?

BLUE SUEDE SHOES - original version

Well, it's one for the money, two for the show, three to get ready, Now go, cat, go

But don't you, Step on my blue suede shoes, well; you can do anything, But lay off of my blue suede shoes

Well, you can knock me down, Step in my face, Slander my name, All over the place

Well, do anything that you want to do, but uh-uh, Honey, lay off of my shoes

93

And don't you, Step on my blue suede shoes, Well, you can do anything, But lay off of my blue suede shoes

VELCRO SHOES - Parkie version

Well, it's one pill at seven, two more at eight, three more at noon, and I still shake

So won't you, Put on my Velcro shoes, Well, I can't do anything, so put on my Velcro shoes

I can't comb my hair, or shave my face; my hands are shaking, all over the place

I used to do anything I wanted to do but uh uh, Honey, help me with my shoes

Please help me; put on my Velcro shoes, I can't do anything, so help me put on my Velcro shoes

Yes, I could have come up with more, but I think you get the picture. Hmm, maybe that wild jerky dancing he did was Parkinson's........ nah, he would have been too young.

Around the World in a Matter of Hours

On Sunday, January 8, 2012, Marie Hamill of our local CBS station, KSWT, interviewed me about my Parkinson's Humor blog. Marie came out to my home and we just talked. She didn't know when it would air, but the producer would notify me. The interview ran locally that same night and I almost missed it; the producer forgot to call and tell me they were going to run it, so I didn't get to tell anyone to watch it.

However, the print version of the story was put on the AP newswire service and by 4 am the next morning, her story about me had spread around the globe and the view counter on my blog was going insane. Here is the print version of the interview:

One local blogger affected by Parkinson's in the Desert Southwest helps thousands of people across the world cope with the disease by using humor. Some call this blogger YumaBev while others call her the jewel in the desert. Her name is Beverly Ribaudo, a year round Yuma resident who has been diagnosed with young onset Parkinson's and writes about her experiences in a comical way. Her blog site is called Parkinson's Humor.

"Instead of telling them the story about me getting stuck in a bath tub, and making it scary, I decided to make it funny. So I told them how the fire men that came to rescue me were all good looking and how I was looking forward to getting a bath everyday, so all the good looking fire men could come and rescue me," says Ribaudo.

Ribaudo says initially she only shared her stories with about 6 people, and they forwarded her blogs to more friends and before she knew it, thousands of people worldwide were logging on and reading her stories.

"It seems like lately I've had a lot of readers from Europe and Eastern Europe, like Russia and it's strange because every time I see a new country, sometimes I have to look it up on a map to see where it is," says Ribaudo.

Ribaudo says she blogs about twice a week but says typing is difficult and can be time consuming for her because of the disease, but says the readers keep her motivated.

"They write to me and they contact me and they tell me that it made them laugh, or that they were having a really bad day and when they read one of my stories it made them feel better. So when you get inspiration like that, it's hard to not keep doing it," says Ribaudo.

Ribaudo is not only a blogger but also a songwriter. Friends of hers say they look forward to karaoke at local bars because Ribaudo writes funny lyrics to sing to common tunes.

Even people who don't suffer from Parkinson's also follow Ribaudo's blog. She says people going through any hard time or just people who need a laugh often read her stories.

Ribaudo encourages any one who is suffering from Parkinson's to join the Yuma Parkinson's support group. The group meets the first Monday of the month.

Marie Hamill, KSWT news

Saying Thank You

Thank You. Those are two words that we use a lot in our daily lives. We say it to strangers who open doors for us, we say it to the person who styles our hair, our neighbors and even our doctors, but how often do you say it to your family?

When is the last time you said Thank You to your spouse, partner, or caregiver and really meant it?

When my Wonderful Husband and I got married 26 years ago, we decided to treat each other as best friends as well as spouses. We never say bad things about each other to anyone and we say Thank You to each other often.

Since this thing called Parkinson's entered our lives, many things have changed, but our appreciation for each other hasn't. He Thanks me for still being able to take care of the laundry and bills and I Thank him for taking out the trash and helping with the floors (both of which were my jobs before PD). I also thank him for cooking (which he is excellent at) and all the other tons of stuff he does.

Neither one of us contemplated that I would be the one who needed taking care of, as I am twenty years younger than him. He never complains and neither do I. I know couples that are in similar situations where the caregiver feels cheated and the one needing care is mean and hateful and yet both of them would never be that way to a friend. It's no ones fault that a serious illness comes into your lives, so don't blame anyone, especially the person you married.

Recently, a neighbor said to my Wonderful Husband that he is amazed at how optimistic I am and last night, my Wonderful Husband said he wondered how life would be if I wasn't. I said, "I hope we never find out." Now, go and say Thank You to your care partner and give them a great big Hug while you are at it.

Thank YOU to everyone who reads this.

A Parkie Goes to the Doctor

I recently went to my family doctor. This was a scheduled visit for a normal check up, nothing urgent, and since my Wonderful Husband's least favorite place to go is a doctor's office, I went alone.

The first thing they did was give me some forms to fill out. I reminded them that I have Parkinson's and that writing is difficult.

Then the nurse called me in and asked me to climb backwards onto a scale so that she could measure and weigh me. (Sure, I thought, no problem, want me to dance a jig, too?)

Next, the nurse handed me a small sterile cup and asked me to give a urine sample and be sure to write my name on the cup. (Sure, I thought, urinate in that tiny cup, maybe. Write my name on it so it can be read, she's got to be joking!) However, off I went.

Urinating in a tiny cup isn't easy for any of us girls, but just try it when you are rigid and your hands are shaking. I managed to get a small amount in the cup and didn't spill any on myself; however, the floor wasn't so lucky.

I was then escorted to the exam room and directed to get undressed and put on a designer "one size fits absolutely no one in the entire world" paper gown and climb up on the table and wait.

By the time the doctor came in, I was laughing almost

99

hysterically. Why? Because we Parkies try to avoid embarrassing or harmful situations and as I sat there, I realized that I had just told a room full of people that I can't write, I could have peed all over myself and maybe broke my neck trying to get weighed.

When I stopped laughing, I told my doctor that visiting her was the most dangerous and humiliating thing I did all week! It turns out she has a sense of humor, too. She said, "Well, at least we know how to dial 911."

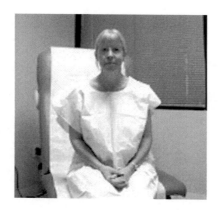

How Do I Describe a Fox to a Cat?

I talked to Cat on the phone. She is my Twitter friend who is blind. Cat had a birthday recently, she is 25 and I am almost 52, but when we talk or Tweet, I don't feel any age difference. Maybe it's because the numbers are the same?

I often wonder what she looks like and I have a picture in my head. Her Mom could send me a photo and then I would know for sure, but even though my "face" is all over the Internet, Cat can only guess what I look like. This makes us even in my book.

Despite the fact that I am old enough to be her Mom and we live on opposite sides of the country and I have Parkinson's and she is blind, we have a lot in common.

We hate it when people feel sorry for us, being blind is normal for her and being a Parkie is now normal for me, so please help us get up if we fall down, but don't feel sorry for us.

We don't understand people who whisper behind our backs, things like "Oh, I think she's blind" or "Look at her arm jerking." Hey, you rude morons, we are NOT DEAF!

We think political correctness has gone too far. She's blind, not visually challenged and I'm a Parkie, not movement challenged.

101

We both have bad days but prefer to laugh them off and have fun and we both sing, though I think she can actually carry a tune.

Cat is curious about Parkinson's and I answer all her questions as best I can. One of the funniest questions she asked me was "Could a person with Parkinson's guide a blind person?" She had read about my dyskinesia and wondered whether a Parkie would be able to steer her safely. I laughed and promised that I would not "guide" her into a telephone pole and that I only wobble sometimes.

One of the hardest questions she asked was "Can you describe what Mr. Fox (Michael J.) looks like?" Now folks, this is the truth, I am the least observant person I know. A good friend shaved his beard off and I did not notice. I don't notice new glasses or haircuts. I can't even tell you what my Wonderful Husband is wearing and I just ate lunch with him sitting right across from me. So, describing Mr. Fox was going to be a challenge.

I found a video of him doing a recent TV guest spot online and I stopped it on a close up of him. I described the shape of his face, nose, mouth and eyes. I said he was short and still looked like a 20-something kid. I described his hair as straight and it was in a normal man's style. She wrote back and said that now she knows exactly what he looks like. It's a good thing, because if I had to describe him right now, to a sketch artist, the drawing might come out looking like Danny Devito.

Cat calls me her Parkie Guide and I like it. The only problem is people keep asking her what kind of dog a Parkie is. I always thought of myself as a cat or a horse, not a dog, but I can bark if needed. Woof!

Happy Birthday Mr. Ali

Dear Mr. Muhammad Ali,

Happy Birthday! I hope you have a great day. You live just a few hours away from me, in Phoenix, Arizona, and I doubt that I will ever meet you, but you are my inspiration. You have never complained about having Parkinson's. You take it in stride and go with the flow. You seem upbeat and have a sense of humor. The way you handle being a Parkie is exactly the way I try to handle it and it is an honor to be included in the same Club Parkinson's as you.

Sincerely yours,

Yuma Bev Ribaudo

A Sturdy New Desk

My Wonderful Husband and I lived and traveled in an RV (recreational vehicle) for sixteen years and the total living space was about 200-square feet, so my computer desk was very small. Everything was small, but we were fine until my strange unknown illness made it difficult to navigate the tight hallways and I could no longer safely drive the truck and tow the RV.

We then moved into a park model RV (a park model is a small manufactured home designed to be set up in an RV park), which has about 400-square feet of living space and my computer desk was still small. I was living here when I finally got diagnosed with Parkinson's and stayed until those tight hallways and entrance steps became problematic.

I now live in a normal size home, but I was still using the tiny homemade computer desk and normally that wouldn't be a problem, but I wobble, I really wobble, and I needed something much sturdier for a desk.

I went shopping and found nothing I liked. The desks were too big or not sturdy enough. The Thrift Store Queen in me took over and I went to my favorite store, The Salvation Army, and found the perfect desk for me. It was real wood, so I bought it and got it home.

I got down on the floor and unhooked all the wires for the computer and everything else in that corner. Why me? Because there are two things that I have always been

105

good at: directions (GPS - 'girl passenger speaks' is a nickname) and wiring (you name it, I can figure out how to wire it so it works). My Wonderful Husband then moved the old desk out and put the new desk in place. It fit, yippee, but it was 8 pm and I was worn out, so I decided to wait until morning to hook everything back up.

Guess what folks? Yup, I was up at 4 am as usual and decided not to wait for my Wonderful Husband to wake up. I wanted to get online and everything was disconnected. I was feeling limber, so I got down on the floor and crawled under the desk and started wiring everything back. Normally, this is a five minute job (keyboard, monitor and mouse), but not in our house. My computer is connected to the usual items, plus a mixer, amplifier, karaoke machine, big flat panel TV, wireless speakers and four regular speakers. My Wonderful Husband and I share a printer, router and modem, and our computers are inter-connected as well, so it looks like wiring for the space shuttle back in that corner!

I got everything hooked up and all the wires nice and neat and it was only 5 am, so I decided to go back to bed. OOPS! I can't get up off the floor; I've been down there too long. I can't even pull myself up using the new desk. Fortunately, I had put the nice thick bathroom rug down to sit on before I started, so I grabbed the pillow off my chair, curled up and went to sleep.

My Wonderful Husband came in later and took a picture of me sleeping under the desk, (he knew it would make a good story), then woke me up, got me up and all was well. He even found a spot for the old desk.

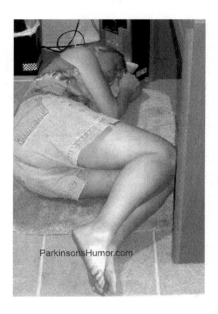

Do I Exercise?

Exercise is a "four letter word" to me and I really don't know how to answer this question when I am asked.

I walk around the house early in the morning standing on my tiptoes with my arms stretched towards the ceiling, but I wouldn't call it exercise. I'm just trying to un-kink all the tightness in my body caused by the Parkinson's and sleeping in the same position all night.

I dance to music, but that's fun, not exercise.

I usually park my car at the far end of the parking lot and grab the nearest cart to help me get to the store, but that's because I don't want the car to get dinged, not for exercise.

At night, while we watch TV, I stretch my arms above my head and out to the side with fingers stretched wide, to un-kink myself before I go to bed, but not for exercise.

I walk every morning with my neighbors, but I don't consider it exercise. We talk and laugh and stop to visit with anyone who is outside, so it's more like a social outing.

I walk from room to room in my house, a LOT, but it's because I can't remember WHY I went into the kitchen, not for exercise.

So, I guess the answer is no, I don't exercise, but I know I should.

I will start tomorrow, I won't have time today, I have to walk with the neighbors, do laundry, go grocery shopping, and I promised my eighty plus something neighbor Erv that I'd teach him how to waltz (he thinks it will help him pick up gals at the senior center) and later is karaoke, but tomorrow, I will start exercising tomorrow, I promise!

Singing for Parkinson's

Monday afternoon is karaoke time for me. Bob & Sylvia host it at a 55+ RV Park not far from my home. I am under 55, but since it is open to the public, I am allowed to join in. I am the only Parkie who comes, but there is a lady with Essential Tremor who also attends, so I am not the only singer with shaking hands.

The people seem to look forward to my silly song parodies and I have done one or two that I wrote about Parkinson's. Bob will usually say "Here comes Yuma Bev, I wonder what surprise she has for us today." Last week I shocked everyone by singing the real words to a song. They clapped, but I think they were a tad disappointed. I will sing my song parodies from now on.

I sing at karaoke for several reasons: It gets me out socially. Too many Parkies hide from people because they are self-conscience. No one has ever said anything mean to me. Most are supportive. Singing is good exercise for our voices. Singing is fun and fun is good for everyone.

No one sings like the professionals do and no one cares that I sing off-key. I have never been booed nor had tomatoes thrown at me. Every one claps for everyone. We dance and Bob puts on silly costumes to fit the song being sung. We laugh and have a great time!

Last week I sang a song about a runaway golf cart and it's based on a true story. Both of my hands were shaking badly, and after, a woman approached me and asked if a music stand would help me. They all now know I have Parkinson's and encourage me, not discourage me.

I advise every Parkie to sing everyday. You don't need karaoke discs, just turn on the radio or type a song you like into an Internet search engine and sing along. Sing loud, sing strong, sing in the shower, or sing while you do laundry. Singing will help you keep the ability to speak. Sing! Sing! Sing!

Besides, it's FUN!

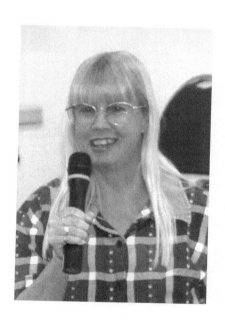

Da Gold Medal

On Friday night, February 3rd, 2012, my Wonderful Husband and I got together with ten of our neighbors and went to our favorite restaurant, Da Boyz, located in downtown Yuma, Arizona. They have excellent Italian food and we go often, usually in a gang of six to twenty.

We made reservations ahead of time and got the Marilyn Monroe room. This room has pictures of Marilyn all over the walls and even a Marilyn deer with fake eyelashes, lipstick and pearls (it's a buck, which makes it even funnier). They have an Elvis room and a Pack Rats room, but I like the dolled up deer (it shows they've got a sense of humor).

I love their lasagna, it's almost as good as my Wonderful Husband makes and I don't have any clean up to do after. I also like their black & white print plates.

Our waiter was a young man named John and I'm not sure he knew what to make of us; we are a pretty silly bunch. I took him aside and told him not to pay attention to anything we said because we just got released from the sanitarium. I think that he might actually have believed me.

Our Gang will throw a party at the drop of a hat. We have had a "Cut the tie off the new Palm Tree" party, a "Got a new dining room table" party, and even a "what the heck, it's the last Thursday of the month" party. If we can't come up with a reason, we'll make something up or drop a hat. My blog reached 10,000 hits a few days before so this was a 10,000 Laughs party (and a good excuse to eat cake)! My friends teased me and they said I looked pretty good for being "hit" so many times and that I was "one tough cookie" for laughing at my Parkinson's.

My Wonderful Husband didn't tell anyone the reason for this party, it was going to be a surprise, but I got surprised instead. My neighbors had decided that I deserved a gold medal and they presented me with one. It was a grand ceremony and even though it was just the logo cut off a sack of flour and glued to a blue ribbon, it meant the world to me and I will treasure it always.

After the presentation, however, I became a big old softy. I tried to tell them how much their friendship meant to me, but I got all choked up and couldn't get the words out, instead tears ran down my cheeks, but I was laughing inside.

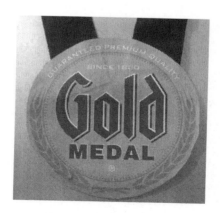

What a Cat Taught a Parkie

Cat is my blind friend that I met through Twitter. She uses screen reader software designed for the blind to "read" what is on her screen. Twitter is her main connection to the outside and she "talks" to people around the world. She is curious, smart, sympathetic, and fun, plus she has a great sense of humor. She willingly answers questions like "How do blind people ...?" as long as they don't get obscene, and she likes to help people as well. When she saw a post about how my fingers stutter when I type, she came up with some great suggestions for Parkinson's people who have trouble typing.

The first one is called Filter Keys and it is a keyboard setting that basically ignores bouncing (trembling) fingers.

The second one is called Sticky Keys and it allows us to hit one key at a time, instead of trying to hit both the Shift and a letter key at the same time to make a capital letter (or Control, Alt, Delete).

The third one is a dictation setting so your computer will type what you speak.

I never knew these settings existed, but apparently they teach blind people about them, and she told me.

If you have XP, the first two can be found in the Accessibility Options part of the Control Panel.

If you have Windows 7, Ease of Access in the Control Panel will lead you to all three settings.

114

Cat also suggested that you look around your home and think what you would change if you were expecting a blind visitor. What's lying around that she might trip over, stumble into or bump her head on? All the things that can hurt her can also hurt a wobbly Parkie and falls can be devastating to all of us.

Everyone should have a Cat for a friend, I'm glad I do.

My Dopamine

I was chatting early one morning and most of us were tired and a little silly. We were discussing possible songs for me to write. Someone said, "Hey, why don't you write a song about dopamine?" Dopamine is the chemical that is missing in our brains. I said, "I can do that, if you help me come up with words that rhyme." So, they started giving me suggestions and I added them to a list of words I was coming up with on my own. The list was becoming longer by the minute and by the time I logged out I had over 30 words. It would be a challenge to use all of them, but I gave it a try. I found the right melody and had to make it longer to accommodate all the extra verses. I had a lot of fun making the music video for this song, managing to find a photo depicting each rhyming word. The tune I used was *Abilene* by George Hamilton and here are the lyrics.

There's a drug called dopamine
It helps me thru my daily routine
Without it I might cause a scene
I gotta take my dopamine

My brain is like an old machine
That's running outta gasoline
And I need something to intervene
I gotta take my dopamine

These shaky hands aren't from caffeine
And I have trouble with fine cuisine
But I can play the tambourine
I gotta take my dopamine

Sometimes I smile like a queen
Other times a wolverine
Most of the time it's in between
I gotta take my dopamine

Sometimes I feel like a latrine
Or that I'm down in a ravine
I keep on fighting like a Marine
I gotta take my dopamine

I zig, I zag and I careen
Like a zombie on Halloween
Or maybe it's more like Charley Sheen
I gotta take my dopamine

Sometimes I sit calm and serene
Sometimes I'm a Mexican Jumping Bean
Every so often I feel like a teen
I gotta take my dopamine

I'd like to be on the silver screen
Or be dancing in a canteen
Other days I don't want to be seen
I gotta take my dopamine

All this movement keeps me lean
I hope these drugs don't hurt my spleen
I have to wear a good sunscreen
I gotta take my dopamine

Sometimes the drugs make me feel green
Or I have trouble getting my teeth clean
It makes it hard to primp and preen
I gotta take my dopamine

Sometimes I'm sad but I'm never mean
Sometimes I'm rigid like a figurine
I hope I never look obscene
I gotta take my dopamine

I wish the experts would convene
And come up with a vaccine
If they find a cure I'll be keen
To wean myself off my dopamine
Until then I'll take my dopamine
My dopamine my dopamine

The Energeezer Parkie

Christine Miserandino wrote a great story called *The Spoon Theory* to explain to her friend what life was like living with Lupus. I have a slightly different way of explaining Parkinson's and use my peculiar sense of humor. I say I'm like the Energizer Bunny, except my battery has Parkinson's and doesn't hold a charge like it should, so I am the Energeezer Parkie.

Everyone has had experience with rechargeable batteries, in cell phones, laptops, cameras, toothbrushes or power tools. We know that when the batteries are brand new and reading 100% charged, they work for days. However, after a while, a 100% charge only gets you half a day or just hours.

This morning, I slept great, woke up feeling good and decided to do the laundry. After the second load was done and the third was in the washer, my battery suddenly died and it was only 10:30 am. It was all I could do to finish the laundry and then I told my Wonderful Husband that I needed to lie down a bit. It was 11:25 am and I asked him to wake me at noon for lunch. I could hear him in the kitchen and I woke up on my own. It was 1:30 pm; I had slept for two hours!

When I asked him why he didn't wake me, he said, "You needed the rest." Now you know another reason why he is the Wonderful Husband.

119

The problem with having Parkinson's is you don't look sick. I wake up almost every morning with my battery reading 100%, but I don't know which battery I got. Did I get the ten-hour battery, the six-hour battery or the two-hour one? I never know. I will never have a brand new battery again and I have accepted it, but when you wake up feeling 100% and then crash three hours later, it makes it difficult to plan your day.

The good news, for me anyways, is that sleep recharges my battery, so a nap can get me through the day.

PS This is the second one of my stories to be featured on the Michael J. Fox Foundation's website. It was a huge honor, to say the least.

The Bendy Toe Blues

My left foot goes crazy almost every day around noon. If I'm walking across a parking lot at the time, it can be a problem. When it does happen, it's called dystonia by the Parkinson's doctors, I just call it cramps.

Sometimes my whole foot tries to turn itself inside out and other times, just my toes curl under. The cramping itself isn't very painful, but my foot doing somersaults inside a shoe is, and trying to walk on it is extremely painful, even barefoot. I usually try to sit down and wait it out. If I catch it soon enough, I can sometimes stand on my tippy-toes and stretch it out or place my bare foot on the cold tile floor (which distracts my brain) and make it go away sooner.

When it happens, I have a hard time getting my shoe off my foot. I am trying to balance on one leg and wrangle a distorted foot out of the shoe. For that reason, I wear oversize boot-type slippers around the house. My feet are small and yet I wear big slippers that make me look like Big Foot. I keep telling you that you've got to have a sense of humor to survive Parkinson's.

Most of my Parkie friends get similar cramps. If they happen first thing in the morning, it's most likely because our brain has run out of medicine while we were sleeping.

121

I used to get painful leg cramps that would jerk me awake. I've mostly ended those by taking my last dose of medicine later and doing specific stretches right before bedtime. I also increased my intake of potassium rich foods.

The foot cramps I get now are most likely caused by too much medicine in one side of my brain. I have Parkinson's symptoms on both sides of my body, but my left side is the least affected and therefore, the muscles get over-stimulated and my foot goes wacky.

I was chatting with other Parkies one day and we were discussing our various foot cramps. Someone suggested that I write a song about our cramping foot blues, so I did.

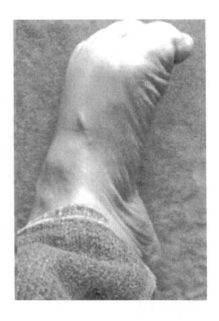

Charting a Parkie, the Results

A few chapters back is a story about how I made a chart of my symptoms for several days prior to a visit with my neurologist. Based on the findings on that chart, we adjusted my medicines. Well, it's been a couple months on the new drug routine and I thought you'd be interested in my results.

I WAS taking a Stalevo 150 and a Requip 1 mg (see Notes below), at 6 am, 2 pm and 10 pm and my chart of symptoms was filled with fives, sixes and sevens and very few tens. (A one is terrible and a ten is very good). I was spending most of the day waiting for the medicines to work. A ten is the best I expect to feel on any given day, not what a ten would be for a person without Parkinson's.

Based on that chart, we decided to lower the strength of the Stalevo and increase the number of times I took it. I NOW take Stalevo 100's at 6 am, 10 am, 2 pm, 6 pm and 10 pm and the Requip 1mg at 6am, 2pm and 10pm (see Notes below). My cell phone alarm goes off to remind me and since it was going off so often, I used some humor and now it plays *I Want a New Drug,* the Huey Lewis song from the 1980's.

I am very pleased with the results and now my chart is filled with mostly nines and tens on an average day.

If there was some way to make today's tens feel like last year's tens, it would be fantastic, but that ain't going to happen. I am worse than I was last year, and much worse than I was two years ago, but I am still doing better than I was the day before I got diagnosed, so life is good, yes very good (and I still feel better after eating chocolate chip cookies)!

Every Parkinson's patient is different and what worked well for me might not work for another patient, and what works well for me today, may not work at all next week. Always consult with your doctor before making any changes to your medications.

Notes:

Stalevo 150 is a brand name combination of 37.5 mg carbidopa USP, 150 mg levodopa USP and 200 mg entacapone

Stalevo 100 is a brand name combination of 25 mg carbidopa USP, 100 mg levodopa USP and 200 mg entacapone

Requip is a brand name of 1 mg ropinirole

Kokopelli

Kokopelli is a mythical figure and his likeness is found all over the southwestern United States. Almost every home in my neighborhood has a Kokopelli symbol on something or the other. I asked my neighbors; most of who are senior citizens, what they thought Kokopelli was known for and they all had the same answer, "Good Luck." That gave me a chuckle.

I had been seeing Kokopelli for years, and I wondered what exactly Kokopelli was all about. After I got diagnosed with Parkinson's, I thought that with his stooped posture that he might have been a Parkie. So, I did what any middle-aged geek would do and I Googled it. Every article I could find on Kokopelli all said the same thing. He was a fertility god; he brought babies to the village maidens.

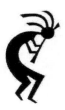

With that knowledge in mind, I began to see just where Kokopelli was featured. There is a casino with a kissable Kokopelli statue featured prominently at the entrance. I guess that's so money reproduces (probably the casinos). There is a Kokopelli likeness at a funeral home (not sure who or what is reproducing there, but I don't want to find out). There are Kokopelli images on ashtrays, coffee

125

mugs, t-shirts, hats, golf balls and even restaurant menus.

So, when I walk around my neighborhood and see all the Kokopelli's, I have to laugh because the only houses that don't have any visible ones are the two houses which actually produced babies in 2011.

Yes, we have a couple Kokopelli's in our home, too. For Good Luck, of course!

Day One of My Vacation from Parkinson's

On Monday, February 27th, 2012, at 4:30 am, I decided to take a vacation. My stepdaughter, Lynn, who is nearly my age, was coming for a visit and I decided that I would NOT have Parkinson's for the four days she would be here.

We left our house at 7 am and drove 182 miles to the four-star resort in Scottsdale, Arizona, where she had spent the weekend on a business trip (she had flown in on Friday from Orlando, Florida). The first 165 miles were easy (nothing but desert and cactus); the last seventeen miles were in big city traffic. She showed us around the resort and treated us to a late breakfast. The service was excellent as was the food, but they had trouble locating a straw for me (I guess most people don't use straws at breakfast). My shaky hands apparently didn't get the NO Parkinson's memo. We left right after eating and headed back home, the first twenty miles were terrifying and stopping for gas was just your average nightmare.

An hour or so later, we stopped in Gila Bend, Arizona and had an ice cream cone, took a bathroom break and snapped a picture of the town's infamous welcome sign. Lynn was beginning to realize that she was in the middle of nowhere and Yuma was only 100 miles farther into nowhere.

We arrived at our house at 3:30 pm and I wanted a nap, but instead, I washed some clothes for Lynn and showed her around our home. At 5:30 pm, we went over to our neighbors for dinner. Sharon made Cornish hens, broccoli and rice pilaf and Freida made Caesar salad and lemon crème cake. I don't know what their husbands did, probably set the table and dug up the extra chairs. Lynn was seated next to me and instantly cut up my hen so that I could eat it (she remembered my troubles with knives).

We sat around gabbing and telling stories and then we played a game where we each drew a picture of a pig and learned all about ourselves from our drawings. My piggy looked like he was doing a wiggle dance. Then I taught everyone how to draw a swan by making a number two and Freida showed us how to draw a three-dimensional box.

Pretty soon it was late (for us) and we drove Lynn to a nice hotel nearby (not a four-star resort, but nice). We decided she'd be more comfortable there, especially with me wandering around the house in the middle of the night.

By the time we got back home, it was 11:30 pm and I was ready for bed. I had been up for nineteen hours. I had survived day one of my Parkinson's vacation.

Day Two of my Vacation from Parkinson's

Tuesday, February 28th, 2012, day two of my vacation from Parkinson's started at 6:40 am, when leg cramps jolted me awake (I guess they didn't get the NO Parkinson's memo). I did my usual morning stuff. We picked Lynn up at her hotel at 10 am and headed for Algodones, a little Mexico border town about ten miles from Yuma, Arizona.

Lynn wanted to look for a new purse, some medicine and jewelry (all available at bargain prices). As we started across the border, my left foot decided to cramp (I guess it didn't get the NO Parkinson's memo either). I figured we'd be out of there by noon, I was wrong. At 2 pm, we found a bakery and had jumbo fresh baked cinnamon rolls for seventy cents each. The only picture I took was one of a little boy riding a dog. It was too crowded to take pictures of her shopping so I found places to sit as Lynn and her Dad shopped.

We wandered around and around and Lynn got right into the bargaining spirit that is the way of life in Mexico. She happily scored a real leather purse, several bracelets and some very nice necklaces for "better than cheap stuff at Wal-Mart" prices and picked up some gifts for friends back at home in Orlando. She bought some antibiotics for her dog and some fancy face cream for herself and her Dad picked up a bottle of Kahlua for a neighbor. It was 4 pm and we decided to leave.

129

Oops, there was a line to get back through the Border and it was FOUR blocks long. We stood in line, well, honestly, Lynn and her Dad stood in line. I would find a bench up ahead and sit down and wait for them to catch up to me and then repeat the process. Most of the people in line had gray hair and were giving me funny looks as I sat, but I didn't care. It took us over two hours to get out of Mexico.

After we finally got back to the U.S.A., we took Lynn to Famous Dave's Bar-B-Que for dinner and then came back to the house. We sat around and visited until 11 pm when we took her back to the hotel.

I had survived day two (kind of).

Day Three of My Vacation from Parkinson's

Wednesday, February 29th, 2012, day three of my vacation from Parkinson's started early, at 5 am with terrible leg cramps again.

Lynn wanted to get some tan while she was here but the weather wasn't cooperating, so I called and made appointments for both of us at Sprayed Rayz to get spray tanned. It would be a "girls" thing. I picked her up at the hotel at 11 am. Neither one of us had ever done this before so I went first. Jonna was patient with me and managed to follow along with my wiggling body (the dyskinesia didn't get the NO Parkinson's memo either) and then it was Lynn's turn. The instructions were to wait six to eight hours before rinsing off even though we looked like we had rolled in mud.

What the heck, Lynn said. I don't know anyone in this town, let's go pick up my Dad and go eat, so we did. He said he'd never had lunch with two pretty mud wrestlers before (ha-ha, his attempt at humor). We ate at our favorite local Italian restaurant, Da Boyz and then we went over to a casino nearby.

Since Lynn was a new casino visitor, they gave her $10 to play with. I'm not sure, but I think she won enough with their money to pay for most of her Mexico treasures. After awhile, it was approaching "rinse the mud off" time so we headed back to the house, stopping to pick up some Subway sandwiches on the way. I rinsed off first and was pleasantly surprised at how natural my new tan looked (not to mention the lack of tan lines, hee-hee). Lynn rinsed off next and she was just as pleased.

We spent our last evening together just sitting around and talking and once again, we took her to her hotel at 11 pm.

I had survived another vacation day from Parkinson's and I was tan, can't get much better than that.

Day Four of My Vacation from Parkinson's (The Final day)

Thursday, March 1, 2012, day four of my vacation from Parkinson's started way, way too early. It was after midnight before I got to sleep and I woke up at 4 am. We didn't need to pick Lynn up until later, so I let my Wonderful Husband sleep in. I played on the computer and started writing this series of stories.

We picked Lynn up at her hotel at 10 am and she and her Dad posed for some pictures, then we headed through the desert towards Phoenix, 200 miles away. We stopped at In-N-Out Burger and grabbed a bite and then fought our way through the traffic and dropped Lynn off at the airport. It was a tearful goodbye for all of us, especially her Dad. Lynn is his only daughter.

I always drive in the big cities because I was born with MapQuest pre-installed in my brain's hard drive. On the way out of the airport, my brain's hard drive froze and I took the wrong exit. I didn't have a map with me, so I had to keep taking exit after exit until I got headed towards home. Needless to say, getting out of Phoenix was a huge nightmare and totally stressed me out. By the time we got to Gila Bend (a town in the middle of nowhere), I had enough. I pulled over and my Wonderful Husband drove the rest of the way home through 100 miles of desert and cactus.

We got home about 5:30 pm and I crashed, I just had to lie down. An hour later, we ate the rest of the subs we'd bought the night before and I put on my pajamas and flopped on the sofa. Lynn called when she got home, which was 9:00 pm our time and I went to bed soon after.

My Wonderful Husband asked me if I missed being around people my own age (Lynn is a few years younger than me) and doing his Daughter's kind of fun. HELL NO was my answer. I may look like I'm in my 30's, but I'm actually 51 and most days I feel like I'm 80 or 90.

The reality is, after my four day vacation from Parkinson's, I still haven't caught up and it's now a week later.

Maybe I need a vacation?

I've still got the tan!

Just Another Day of Parkinson's

I was wide-awake early one morning, as usual. There was no one online so I decided to mop our floors. As I was mopping, I started composing lyrics to a new song. By the time the sun came up, I had written, recorded and made the music video to Just Another Day of Parkinson's. I picked the country song *There Ain't Nothing Wrong with the Radio* for the melody and here are the lyrics.

In bed at eleven, up at four
Thought up these words, as I mopped the floor
Before 6 am, this song will be done
Just another day of Parkinson's

I checked the email, did Facebook
Gave the news, a quick look
Sent a couple tweets, just for fun
Just another day of Parkinson's

There's a whole bunch of pills that I take
I want to eat breakfast, but I have to wait
My hands aren't steady sometimes they shake
But I don't worry about the things I break
I pick up the pieces, grab the glue gun
Just another day of Parkinson's

My fingers stutter, when I type
And it's even worse, when I write
The bank says they can't tell my three from a one
Just another day of Parkinson's

I find myself stumbling, when I walk
And if my foot cramps, I have to hop
It's a good thing I don't have to run
Just another day of Parkinson's

I like to dress fancy, look real nice
When I buy clothes, I gotta think twice
Tiny little buttons, give me the blues
And I only wear Velcro shoes

But I keep shopping, I'm having fun
Just another day of Parkinson's
I keep laughing, I'm having fun
Just another day of Parkinson's

For this video I used pictures to illustrate the lyrics. My
Wonderful Husband couldn't believe that I took a picture
of myself, in my pajamas, mopping the floor and put it
online for the world to see. "Its funny!" was all I said.

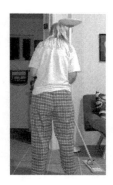

Reflections of Me at 25 and 52

Today, March 8th, 2012 is my 52nd birthday. I woke up at 4:44 am and I was born at 4:44 pm. I started thinking about my 25th birthday and how much my life changed that one-year.

I spent most of my 25th birthday alone and crying. The boy I was dating had dumped me the night before and then everyone forgot my birthday. Everyone. I didn't blame them; my Moomer had died six weeks earlier, so no one was thinking about me. Life was awful, my first husband had died in a fiery car crash two years earlier and then I watched my Mom slowly die of lung cancer. I wished I were dead, too.

My Mother came to visit me in a dream that night. She scolded me and told me to shape up and get on with my life. It was very real, like she was standing right there, so I went to counseling, gave up my apartment and moved back home with my Dad, found a new job and started taking some college classes.

A couple months later I ran into a male friend that I hadn't seen in many years. Our friendship took up right where it left off. We enjoyed being together. One day, I asked this friend if he would ever consider marrying me. He said yes, but thought we should at least date first. We did. We got engaged on July 24th and married on December 14th, 1985.

137

My Wonderful Husband and I have been together ever since then. My 25th year started out in tears and ended in love.

Tonight will be a full moon; my 25th birthday was also on a full moon. I went outside early this morning and snapped pictures of last night's moon as it was setting. I don't remember seeing the moon years ago, but I am sure I did.

As I came back towards the house (in my pajamas, slippers and with two coats on), a terrific sight greeted me as I walked up to my door. My neighbors had gone to the trouble of making a "Happy Birthday Bev!" banner and hung it on my porch. I don't know when they did it, but it must have been very early.

When I turned on my computer and checked my emails, Twitter and Facebook, there were lots of birthday wishes. At 8 am, I climbed back into bed and snuggled up to my Wonderful Husband. I think that this year is going to be a very good one.

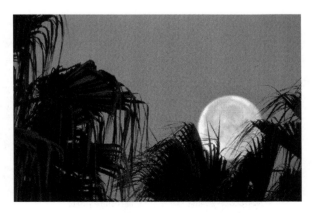

My Birthday Was GREAT!

I woke up early on my Birthday and wrote the previous story about the first few hours of my 52nd Birthday and then went back to bed.

You might be wondering about the rest of the day. The rest of the day was great!

The neighborhood jeeping gang sang to me before they took off for the day and of course, there was the big banner across my porch. I acted surprised when I saw it with Hubby and the neighbors.

My Twitter and Facebook accounts were full of Happy Birthday wishes as were my email and regular mailboxes.

George and Freida, my walking buddies, treated us to lunch and then I had a little nap. After dinner, we went over to George and Freida's house for cake. Freida is an excellent baker and while I normally do not like cake, she has managed to make one that I LOVE. It tastes like cinnamon rolls and Snicker doodle cookies, both of which I love. Willie and Sharon were there as well. I got to blow out candles while everyone sang Happy Birthday to me.

Everyone complimented me on the sweater that I was wearing. My Wonderful Husband gave me that sweater the first year we were married. Yes, it was 26 years old!

It was, definitely, one of the best Birthday's I've ever had.

139

Farm-a-college-ee of Parkinson's

Reading all the fine print on those fact sheets that come with Parkinson's medications is confusing and boring, so I decided to use humor to try to explain it. I got the idea of using farm references by the phonetic pronunciation of Pharmacology (FARM-a-college-ee).

Parkinson's is caused when certain neurons in our brain die and quit producing dopamine. Low dopamine levels cause the signals from our brain to our muscles to get scrambled and produces the erratic movements. Okay, just give us dopamine. The solution sounds simple, but there is a catch: our bodies are very protective of what it lets in the barn (brain) and dopamine can't even get on the farm.

The scientists developed levodopa, which can get on the farm, but by itself, levodopa causes intense nausea and vomiting and turns into dopamine and still can't get in the barn (brain). The scientists found that by adding carbidopa to the levodopa, they could prevent it from becoming dopamine and quell the nausea. Carbidopa is like a Judas Goat; it leads the levodopa past the guard dogs and right into the barn (brain). The brand name combination of carbi/levodopa is called Sinemet.

The problem with Sinemet is that our bodies try to get foreign items out of our bloodstream. It takes about 45 - 75 minutes from mouth to blood stream and then our efficient blood cleansing organs get rid of it about an hour later, so not much makes it into the barn (3%

according to the experts).

The scientists went back to work and found out that if they added another drug called entacapone (Comtan), they could keep the Sinemet in our bloodstream longer and therefore more can be herded in to the barn known as your brain. The brand name combination of Sinemet and Comtan is called Stalevo.

Comtan has an astonishing side effect of making your urine turn bright yellow, orange or even brown. This has a tendency to freak out the lab techs when they ask you to pee in a cup. It is my own personal observation that this yellow stain also creeps into your saliva and perspiration and I am pretty sure that it is staining my teeth as well (just call me mellow yellow).

There is another class of drugs called dopamine agonists. These drugs aren't designed to replace the missing dopamine; they are designed to make the receptors that use dopamine work better without it. It's kind of like dangling a carrot in front of a donkey.

There are 2 main agonists: Ropinirole and pramipexole, known under the brand names of Requip and Mirapex. These drugs do such a good job of stimulating the receptors that they can cause dangerous obsessive or compulsive behaviors such as gambling, uncontrollable shopping or risky sexual activity. IF you are taking an agonist, you need to be aware of these potentially life altering side effects and find someone you can trust to monitor you. On the up side, agonist's have also been tied to increased creativity. People start writing poetry or

141

take up painting when they had no interest prior.

Rasagiline (Azilect) and selegiline (Eldepryl) are other drugs that are used in Parkinson's and are in a class of medications called monoamine oxidase (MAO) type B inhibitors. They work by increasing the amounts of certain natural substances in the brain and act similar to the agonists. They are often prescribed to recently diagnosed Parkies in an attempt to delay prescribing the Sinemet.

There are many other drugs used to either treat the symptoms of Parkinson's or the side effects of the drugs we take to relieve our symptoms.

Treatment of Parkinson's consists of easing our symptoms only. None of the currently available medications will stop the progression or cure it. Over time, Sinemet causes unpleasant side effects and becomes less effective, requiring us to take higher and higher doses, so doctor's try to reduce the amount we take or delay its usage.

The reason Sinemet loses its effectiveness is the brain needs healthy dopamine producing neurons to convert the levodopa into dopamine, and, as the disease progresses, there are less and less neurons to do the converting.

We Should Be Dancing

I love to dance, I have always loved to dance and having Parkinson's isn't going to stop me from dancing. Dancing uses a different part of your brain than walking, so it is very beneficial for people with Parkinson's to dance (and it's fun).

Back in the late 70's, my dance partner Dwayne and I used to enter (and often win) dance contests around central Florida. We were a good team and used to do some pretty spectacular lifts and tricky routines. I wore skimpy costumes, high heels and felt like a dancing queen.

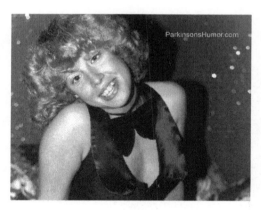

In the early 80's, my competition days ended and Dwayne and I went our separate ways. I got married, became a widow, got married again, but I still liked to dance. Line dancing became popular in the 90's, no partner was needed and I soon mastered all the dances, including the ones with tricky footwork. Of course, what I really liked was the cowboy hat!

Now it's 2012 and my feet aren't coordinated enough to do the fancy steps, but I still put on old disco tunes or a country song and shuffle around to the beat. I like it! It makes me feel like that dancing queen from 30+ years ago and maybe; just maybe, it will help me maintain my balance and my ability to walk for many more years to come.

So, friends, put on some music and dance, dance, dance. Use some humor; put on The Shake (Sam Cooke), Shake Your Booty (KC & Sunshine Band), Shake Your Body (Michael Jackson), Country Girl Shake it for Me (Luke Bryan), The Shake (Neal McCoy), Shake It Up (The Cars) or Walk Like An Egyptian (The Bangles).

A Parkie Hospital Kit

When I first heard about the National Parkinson Foundation's Aware in Care Kit, designed to help Parkinson's patients get the best possible care when hospitalized, I ordered one right away and then I shared the ordering information on my Facebook and Twitter pages.

My kit came in a few weeks. I looked it over and decided it was important, so I showed it to my neighbor, Carole, who volunteers at our local hospital as a patient advocate. She ordered one and plans to talk about the kit at the next hospital board meeting. I told all the people at my local Parkinson's support group about the kit and helped eighteen of them order kits for themselves. It's a good thing my neighbor is warning the hospital because I am certain these kits will be appearing with Parkies coming in for treatment.

The kit is small, but packed with useful information. Here are the contents of the kit:

1. The Hospital Action Plan brochure: It has great advice about planning ahead for your next hospital stay, emergency or planned. Hint: Make sure that everyone knows EXACTLY WHERE the nearest hospital or care center is located, before an emergency comes up because getting lost on your way isn't funny. Make sure you can FIND your kit in an emergency; I keep mine next to my coffee cup, because I ALWAYS know where my coffee cup is.

145

2. The Medical Alert Card: This should be filled out and carried in your wallet at all times. Hint: Have someone who can write legibly fill it out for you. It won't help you if the Emergency responders can't read your scribbled writing.

3. The Parkinson's Disease Medical Alert Bracelet: This gave me some trouble. I have difficulty with clasps, so I could NOT put it on by myself. My Wonderful Husband (a former jeweler) solved the problem by shortening the links and making it just loose enough that I can slide it on without unhooking it. The front of it says to look for the wallet card and the back of it has a 1-800 number for Parkinson's info.

4. Medication Form Pad: This is a whole pad of forms to list your medications and exactly what time you take them, so update it each time you have ANY changes. Hint: It might be a good idea to have someone else fill this form out, too. I have one in my kit and copies in the glove boxes of both family cars, just in case I don't have the kit with me if an emergency comes up.

5. Magnet: Use this magnet, in the hospital, to display a copy of your Medication Form. It will stick right to the end of the bed where your chart hangs.

6. Parkinson's Disease Fact Sheet: A simple explanation about Parkinson's and how IMPORTANT it is for us to get the right medications at the right times during our hospital stay, as well as warnings of medications that can have potentially bad side effects. Hint: I made copies of mine and gave one to each of my doctor's to put in my

146

chart and I also put a copy in each car's glove box.

7. The "I have Parkinson's" Reminders Slips are to be given to EVERY person who will be taking care of you in the hospital.

8. A Thank You Card: To give to the staff member who did their best to give you high quality care. Hint: the one you'd give an A+ to. (Not the prettiest or handsomest one, give them your phone number instead, hee-hee)

Hopefully, I won't ever need to use my kit, but just in case, I think I'll be able to squeeze my stuffed Parky Penguin (a gift from Shirley) and my pajamas in the kit along with a toothbrush and comb.

Just in case the nurses are a bit grumpy, my pajamas (black & white prison stripes with Alcatraz Reject stamped across the front in bright red) ought to give them a smile, at least.

Go to www.awareincare.org to order yours today. Sorry, but it can only be sent to U.S.A. addresses. I almost forgot the most important thing; these kits are FREE, yes FREE, so order yours right now.

Attention Non U.S.A. Readers: If you go to the website and click Kit Contents, most of the forms are down loadable, so you can print them out and make your own kit.

According to Rush

In March 2012, Michael J. Fox appeared on CNN. The remarks made by Rush Limbaugh calling Mr. Fox's excessive Parkinson's movements "fake" was brought up again. Mr. Fox said as a celebrity, those kinds of remarks were just part of the job. However, as a non-celebrity Young Onset Parkinson's patient, I felt as though Rush was calling me and every other Parkie out there fakes as well.

I wrote my own response to Rush Limbaugh in the form of a poem and then recorded myself reciting the poem. Here is the poem:

According to Rush

Whenever we watch a Mike Fox interview
My husband says "It's just like watching you"
He says I do the same wiggle and shake
According to Rush, I must be a fake

Some parts of the day I can barely move
Other times my body does a jerky groove
It's like having my own earthquake
According to Rush, I must be a fake

I have trouble just signing my name
And buttoning buttons is not a fun game
I have to have someone else cut my steak
According to Rush, I must be a fake

My feet shuffle when I walk
And some times I drool when I talk
The medicines make me move like a snake
According to Rush, I must be a fake

My face is almost frozen in a blank stare
But I can still look into the camera there
And because I did this in just one take
According to Rush, I must be a fake

If Rush would spend a day in my shoes
I bet he'd be singing the Parkinson's blues
But Rush as a Parkie would be a mistake
According to Rush, he would be a fake

It's bad enough that sometimes our doctor's think we are faking symptoms, when all we want is answers. Some Parkies have been told by their employers and their own families they are faking. We are not faking anything. Trust me, if I could stop the movements, I would, but I can't and people calling us a fake is just not right.

Parkinson's Awareness Month - Getting Displays in My Local Library

I ordered pamphlets from the Parkinson's Disease Foundation (PDF) and then talked to Iris, the manager of my local branch Library about setting up a display for Parkinson's Disease Awareness Month (April). She loved the idea and she suggested that I talk to someone at the Main Library, which I did, and they said they'd be happy to do something county wide, so I gave all the pamphlets to Iris to take to the next managers meeting.

WOW! Yesterday I went in to my local branch and Iris had set up a beautiful display. I had my camera with me and I snapped a few pictures and sent them to the PDF.

Later in the day, I stopped in at the Main Library and they had set up an outstanding display as well.

It was easy; I ordered materials and then asked my library to set up a display. I bet you could get your local library to do the same thing.

Does Parkinson's Hurt?

Most medical doctors will say Parkinson's doesn't hurt, but they don't HAVE Parkinson's. Hmmm, a neurologist with Parkinson's, that would be humorous, unless he does brain surgery! The actual process of the neurons dying off in our brains is painless, however, the strange things Parkinson's makes our limbs and body parts do, CAN cause pain.

Foot cramps are painful, no doubt about that! Tremors are painful for our family and friends to watch and are a big pain in the butt for us Parkies, but don't usually hurt, unless we spill hot coffee down the front of our shirt. Ouch!

My rigidity is usually painless, but very aggravating. I generally have two or more bruises on my arms or legs from bumping into doorways because I zigged when I should have zagged or from getting up awkwardly from the desk or table. They hurt, but can you say that it's Parkinson's? If I fall and break my leg, can I blame Parkinson's? What about back pain from being stuck in the same position all night?

I say YES, absolutely YES! All kinds of things in life hurt. Giving birth to a baby hurts, but women have more than one. The death of your parents or spouse hurts. A hangover hurts, but many people don't quit drinking. The reality is life, in general, involves some pain.

151

When I am having a bad day, I ask myself "Have you ever felt worse than this?" If the answer is YES, then I say to myself "Then what are you complaining about?" then I laugh and instantly feel better. If the answer is NO, then I have something to compare the next bad day with.

Yes, I do argue with myself and sometimes, I win the argument.

Yuma Arizona Proclaims April as Parkinson's Awareness Month

On Monday, April 2nd, 2012, both the Yuma County Board of Supervisors and the City of Yuma proclaimed April as Parkinson's Awareness Month. I wish I could say I was the architect, but I wasn't. I sent emails to everyone, but my local Parkie friend Greg Gardner made it happen.

Greg is our local support group leader and has been a Yuman for many, many years. He worked in local radio before Parkinson's forced his "retirement" and knows every politician in our community. I, on the other hand, am a fairly recent Yuman and until last Monday, had never met any of our local politicos.

The Board of Supervisor's met at 9 am and Greg and I received the official Proclamation together.

Our support group was meeting at noon and Mayor Alan Krieger of Yuma joined us for lunch and officially presented the City's Proclamation.

After reading the Proclamation, Greg and the Mayor turned to me and said we'd like to present this Proclamation to Bev Ribaudo, for all the work she does for Parkinson's. It was an emotional moment for me and I could barely squeak out "Thank you."

Board member Lenore Stuart also joined us for lunch and presented the County Proclamation to our group.

153

We had a great lunch and the best desserts and Greg told the Board of Supervisor's that the reason he was wearing yellow was because he was the top banana of our group.

All in all, it was a great day for Parkinson's.

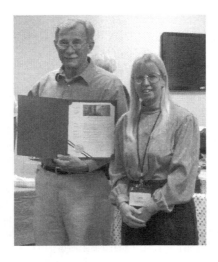

Mayor with Proclamation

David and Me

David is my brother. He is three years older and had bad luck before he was even born. Mom had pneumonia during her pregnancy and David got the mumps and measles when he was just weeks old. My grandmother didn't pay attention when she was changing his diaper and he rolled off the table. He fell (or got pushed) off a two-story building, fell off a motorcycle, got severe burns on his feet and got hit by a car.

When Mom was seven months pregnant with me, she was told David was retarded and her age was probably a factor (she was 38 when he was born) and that the current baby (me) would probably be worse. I was born with a cold, but other than that, I was normal. The doctors told Mom to put David in an institution, but she said NO, he belonged at home.

I didn't know David was different until I got in grade school, when other kids called him names and threw rocks at him. Their parents weren't much better; they wouldn't let their children come to our house because he was different. I guess they thought their kids might "catch it". Who would have thought adults could be so dumb?

David was my playmate growing up. He liked Tonka trucks and I hated dolls, so we got along fine, playing in the dirt. I fought the jerks that teased and bullied him because no matter what they did to him, he wouldn't fight back. Most of David's problem was speech related,

155

he understood exactly what you said to him but, when he tried to reply, the words got all garbled up on the way out. He laughed at good jokes and managed some simple one-syllable words, his favorites being Coke and truck, though it came out more like coe and truh, but I understood him.

When I was about six, Mom said she wished someone would teach David how to pee standing up and since I had taught him to tie his shoes and write his name with a crayon, I thought she was talking to me. She wasn't, but I didn't know that! While playing in the woods across the street from our house, I had to go and having seen little boys do it, I tried it myself. Then I showed David. He was much better at it than I was and Mom just laughed when I proudly told her what I had done.

David had seizures in his sleep. I was about seven the first time I awoke and saw one. Mom showed me how to hold his head to the side until it was over. Many nights, I was the only one who heard him. I guess I should have been scared, but Mom made it seem normal, so I never was.

Nothing ever seemed to bother David. Oh, he got frustrated some times when people couldn't understand what he wanted, but usually he would figure out a way to make them understand. He was fearful of little kids and small yapping dogs, but could approach the most vicious big dogs and they would wag their tails and snuggle up to him. Cats seemed to have affection for him, too. David was always happy, laughing or smiling.

Once, when we were adults, during Thanksgiving dinner at my home, a drink got knocked over. Everyone panicked, except David. He grabbed his napkin and mopped it up, even though he wasn't the one who spilled it. Then he gave a hearty laugh and grabbed some more turkey! Now, tell me, who was the smart one?

I have a special place in my heart for anyone who is different and my Parkinson's seems minor compared to David's life. I taught David how to tie his shoes and pee like a man, but he taught me how to LIVE and LOVE and most of all ...LAUGH!

The Funny Cactus

I saw the cactus last summer on one of my morning walks, and took a picture of it and laughed when I saw it on my computer. I made a humorous Parkinson's cartoon out of it.

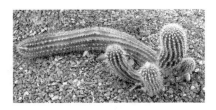

A month later, it bloomed and it was even funnier.

I met the owner, Bill, last fall and told him about his cactus and its funny bloom. He told me the story of how he acquired it. He said it was over in the corner of the cactus place, almost hidden from view. It had been a nice cactus, but the wind had knocked it over and now it was ruined. Bill saw it and asked "How much?" and the man said "$5, you can cut the main stem off and the rest will grow fine," so Bill took it home and planted the whole thing, fallen stem and all and then he went home to Canada for the summer. He said everyone called it the Viagra cactus and teased him about it.

I promised to email him a photo if it bloomed again while he was gone this summer.

Well, the funny cactus did bloom again, twice, since Bill left. The first time was in March and I took a picture of it that I entered in a contest (I didn't win).

The second time was just a few days ago and it was stunning.

I guess the funny cactus had the last laugh. All it needed was someone to overlook its imperfections, take it home, treat it well and let it shine. Don't we all?

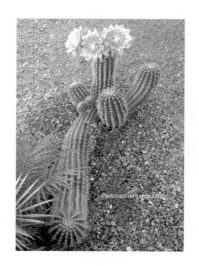

Where's the Cake?

I received a message from the Michael J. Fox Foundation on Friday, April 6, 2012.

It turns out the folks at 23andme (a genetic testing company looking for bio-markers for Parkinson's) found some surprising associations. One of them was that people with Parkinson's have a tendency to develop a sweet tooth.

The story piqued my interest and I began thinking about my own sweet tooth.

I was a strange child. I did not like sweets. My parents loved sweets. My siblings did, too. When we bounded in the door after school, the others grabbed a handful of cookies and I grabbed a chunk of cheese. I used to joke that by the time I was born, all the sweet tooth genes were gone. This made my birthday celebrations tricky for my Mother, who was an exceptional baker. I did not like cake or pie and I really didn't even care for ice cream, so Mom would improvise. She'd put candles in cubes of cheese, in slices of apple or sticking out of the bowl of mashed potatoes. My favorite memory was when she made a fancy jello ring, only it didn't quite set firm enough and the candles slowly fell over the sides on the way to the table.

My lack of interest in sweets continued into adulthood, I only ate a bite or two of my own wedding cake and I still prefer cheese.

160

In the last couple of years, things have changed. I find myself coming back from the buffet with desserts on my plate instead of fruit and salad. Unless it's chocolate, which I still don't like, I will even eat birthday cake with ice cream at parties. I've begun to eagerly look forward to my neighbors making holiday cookies and my walking buddy Freida, hasn't made one dessert yet that I didn't want a second piece of.

What is going on with me? Has my sweet tooth gene finally awakened after 50 years?

Apparently not, I can blame it all on Parkinson's. Yes, it's all Parkinson's fault.

Now, I have a question for the researchers. My sweet tooth only started AFTER I started taking medications for the Parkinson's. I had no sweet tooth for the eight plus years that I was searching for a diagnosis. So is the sweet tooth caused by the Parkinson's or just another strange side effect of the medications we take?

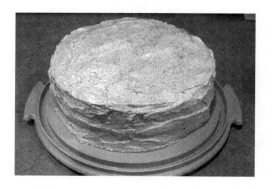

Dr. Z and Me

I went to see Dr. Z, my neurologist, on Wednesday, April 18, 2012. Going to see Dr. Z is like visiting a friend, I have been seeing him every two or three months since August of 2007, when he first diagnosed me with Parkinson's.

My visits always start the same, Bonnie or Malinda sign me in, then Perla shows us (my Wonderful Husband always comes along) to an exam room and in few minutes, Dr. Z comes in, smiles a big smile, and says "Hello, how are you today?"

Part one of my visit was as his patient. He asked me how I was doing with the dosing changes we made last visit (three months ago). I told him I was having bad left foot cramps (my lesser affected side) everyday around noon (during peak on time) and that I had tried cutting back my Stalevo 100's to four times a day (after Charting my symptoms) instead of five, to see if it made a difference. The foot cramps had disappeared and the slight increase in off time was acceptable to me, so he wrote down the new dosing times and said okay.

We then discussed the possibility of replacing a couple of the Stalevo's with plain Sinemet (I am concerned about the potential negative side effects of the higher doses of entacapone, the extra ingredient in Stalevo). Dr. Z said I could try it, but do it slowly and carefully chart my symptoms. He said I might need to take a half pill in between doses and wrote me a prescription. I asked

162

I asked, meekly, about the "spots". She said the one on my nose was vascular (probably blowing your nose too much from allergies), she said the one on my arm was just "your skin getting old and sun damage" and she called the one on my neck a keratosis or barnacle.

She said everything was fine; she'd see me in six months and disappeared. I got dressed and found myself singing *Barnacle Bill the Sailor Man* the rest of the day! I was a very Happy Parkie, even though she said I was old and had barnacles like an old ship! But my nose was spared the scalpel once again. Whew!

Mention of melanoma risk is in the fine print of Stalevo, Sinemet, Requip and Mirapex, all of which I have taken during my treatment of Parkinson's.

Joy and Sorrow, Worries and Cheers

The week of April 23, 2012, was a mix of emotions for both my Wonderful Husband and me.

On Monday, we celebrated Freida's birthday. Phil & Ruth invited all of us for lunch; we had cake and spent the afternoon laughing. Freida had trouble blowing out the candles, but managed to blow most of the cinnamon sugar off the cake and all across the table. We were all giggling like a bunch of teenagers.

On Tuesday, we attended a Celebration of Life service for a friend who passed away suddenly. David's death was quite a shock; we had just seen him a few days earlier. I was concerned the emotional toll might exaggerate my Parkinson's symptoms and make me stand out in the crowd, but I did okay.

On Thursday, I went to the dermatologist, I was worried, but everything was fine.

On Friday, we went to see a local high school play and cheered at the very good acting.

It was a week of emotional ups & downs and I took extra naps, but I lived my life and did NOT let Parkinson's ruin it. Good advice for all of us.

This Parkie Takes a Picture

I like to take pictures, but since I have Parkinson's, I am not exactly steady. I have an inexpensive point & shoot camera with a viewfinder as well as the display screen. Holding the camera against my face helps and it has image stabilizer built in, which means it will adjust for some movement (shaky hands, wobbling body). I should use a tripod, but I'm too lazy, and I'd probably knock the whole thing over.

My neighbor, Sharon, is a Master Gardner, so her yard is a favorite place for me. She has blooming plants, interesting decorations and an unobstructed view of the mountains to the east. She finds humor in the blonde girl, still in pajamas, wandering in her yard, taking photos at sunrise.

My photos of her cactus blooms have been featured in my blog stories. I even won a Facebook flower photo contest with one. The prize was a worm farm (no, I don't know what it is), which I promptly donated, sight unseen, to the local 4H club.

The nice people at the University of Arizona - Cooperative Extension Department contacted me recently and asked permission to use a different one of my cactus pictures for their brochure. They offered me a signed book on *Arizona Insects* by Carl Olson as compensation. I guess I should have kept the worm farm; I could have fed the worms to all the insects I can now identify. I, of course, said YES and promptly called and told Sharon the news.

Well, the insect book and a sample of the brochures arrived. I was expecting the little 4x8 type flyer found in hotel lobbies. Instead, it was a big tri-fold fancy brochure and right inside was my photo, prominently featured. Needless to say, I was thrilled.

Then I looked closer and there it was, in small print, "Photo by YumaBev." Photo credit was a bonus; it wasn't part of the deal.

So, now I guess I can add photographer right after humorist and songwriter on a resume'. Of course, no one will be able to read my handwriting except maybe a doctor or pharmacist.

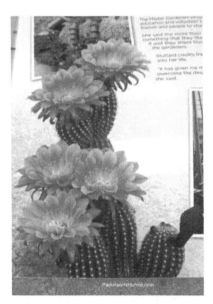

Support Groups Are Fun

I go to a local Parkinson's support group, but a lot of my Parkie friends won't go to these meetings. They say it is too depressing, seeing people who are worse off then they are. I think they are wrong.

I am the youngest Parkie in my group, but younger people do come to learn how to help Mom or Grandpa. We have members in all stages of this disease and the one thing I have noticed is: we all look forward to these once-a-month lunchtime gatherings. Why? We share stories, we laugh, we see how people have adapted, we see hope, and of course, the desserts are great!

There are a few who still work for a living, which I cannot. There are a few who have had the DBS (Deep Brain Stimulation) surgery and there are some who can no longer walk, but we all connect with one another, plus our care-partners get to talk to other care-partners and there are a lot of hugs.

The way I see it, if seeing other Parkies in worse shape than you are is depressing, then I guess you shouldn't go visit your Parents when they get older and forget the Grandparents completely. After all, they aren't young anymore and you will probably end up looking like one of them someday. I already have the "Goshert" family chin, so prominent in family photos of my Aunts, Uncle and Grandpa.

Maybe it's because I grew up with senior citizen parents,

but I like being around older people. Most don't complain about what they can't do anymore. Joke about it? Yes. Laugh about it? Yes, but complain? No.

Plus, they have unique ways of adapting, like the man I saw yesterday using his golf putter as a cane, "Works much better this way than it ever did on the golf course!" he said. Or the one that had all his buttons on his favorite shirts replaced with snaps "I can pretend I'm a Chippendale at bed time and just rip it open!" he laughed.

Check out a local support group, if there is one near you, you might just have a good time and make some new friends! Plus the desserts are really, really good.

Driving My Life Away

People are surprised to learn I drive. I was and still think I am, a good driver. As soon as I got my license at age sixteen, my parents handed me the keys every time we went anywhere. I was the only non-employee allowed to drive my husband's company car. I have driven everything from a very tiny car to a 34-foot motor home, automatic transmissions and stick shifts, and I've towed boats, campers and big 5th wheels. I have never been in an accident and never get tickets. I am the annoying person who uses turn signals and drives the speed limit.

There are other reasons I drive.

1. I don't like to ride, and if I close my eyes in a car, I get car sick (no sleeping for me either).

2. It is easier for me to get in and out of the driver's seat, because my left leg works better than the right one. I guess I won't be driving in those countries where you sit on the right side of the car (looks like England and Australia are spared).

3. I have an exceptional sense of where I am and where I need to get. I can usually just glance at a map and then find my way there. I joke that I came with MapQuest installed in my brain.

Now, if my Wonderful Husband also liked to drive, we'd have a problem, but unless it's a convertible with the top down, he'd rather be a passenger, so we're good for now. In fact, I drive so much of the time; people assume my

171

Wonderful Husband doesn't drive. I have driven in 49 of our 50 states and most of the lower Canadian Provinces. I did, actually, have my hands on the tiller of a cruise ship in Alaska, but the Captain wouldn't let me drive it.

My Car Shopping Adventure

I was having trouble getting out of our car due to Parkinson's. Getting IN was fine, but getting OUT was becoming difficult and even though it was a luxury car (an older one); the seats were becoming uncomfortable for me. We had a second car, a convertible, but it was even harder for me to get out of.

I have about an hour every morning when I can move like a normal person, almost, so I decided to go car looking. I say looking because I was doubtful that I would find the right car for me.

We have all the big brands in our town and all the dealers are in a row, so I started with the bigger SUV types, thinking that higher off the ground would be better. They were easy to get OUT of, but not so easy to climb IN to. I am on the short side, barely 5 foot 2, and these are for tall Papa Bears, not this little Goldilocks.

My biggest obstacle, at the car places, was that I don't LOOK like there is anything wrong with me, so the salesmen kept asking what color and what options I wanted and they were confused when I would say, "I just want one that fits me."

My Wonderful Husband said, "Let's look at the sporty models." So, I tried them, they looked sharp, but I needed the salesman's help to get out. These cars are designed for middle age Guy Bears, not me. We ruled out the sedans (since the two in our garage weren't right for

173

me) and I didn't want a Mama Bear mini-van. I tried the smaller SUV types, but nothing fit. Every vehicle we tried was either hard to get in to or hard to get out of.

I could only try a few each day, before I got too rigid, and I was just about to give up when I saw a used PT Cruiser. I gave it a try, and it FIT. Perfectly! It was easy to get in and out of, plus it had an armrest that moved with the seat and a place for my purse. I could reach the pedals without being up against the steering wheel and the color was beautiful, but best of all, it was a convertible (a Wonderful Husband Bear thing), and so we bought it.

Goldilocks and her handsome prince "Cruise" happily ever after.

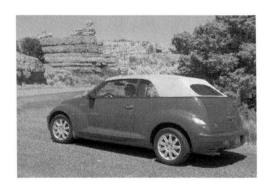

It Was a Serious Day for Me

Things in my neighborhood got serious this morning, seriously Cereus. Seven different Cereus cactus plants bloomed early today. Three were in Carole's yard (she lives next door) and four were in Sharon's yard (she lives next to Carole). I knew last night some would bloom but I was pleasantly surprised when ALL of them did. I must have taken fifty photos to get good ones of each (even with image stabilization, a lot of my shots are blurry). The first one opened around 5 am and the last one waited until almost 9 am (I guess even cacti sleep in). It was a stunning display of color, but only a few people got to see them in real life. Even their owners will only get to see them in photos. The flower show didn't last long, by 4 pm; all of them were closed up. See, there is something good about Parkinson's, I wake up early and get to see beautiful things like this. Life is good.

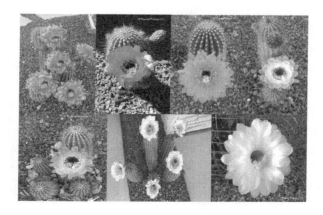

175

Will Parkinson's Kill Me?

The short answer is NO, you will die WITH Parkinson's not of Parkinson's, or so I am told. I'm not going to worry about it since I might get run over by a truck next week or go to the dentist.

My Dad was diagnosed with Parkinson's when he was 82 and he also had some dementia, but it was a trip to the dentist or eating lunch that probably killed him. He was doing great; we went to the dentist and the podiatrist and then out for lunch. He was climbing in and out of the car better than I could. Less than 24-hours later, he was in the hospital with a high temperature, a virus of some kind. The virus knocked the heck out of him and the folks at the hospital didn't help any. They wanted him to stay in bed, but he kept forgetting and he would get out of bed to use the bathroom, so they secured him and he fought back. They asked me to bring his wheel chair, I said, "He doesn't have one, yesterday he was walking better than I am.", but they didn't believe me.

The day before, we had eaten a nice lunch at a casual restaurant and Dad had no problems swallowing his food, but the folks at the hospital insisted on a swallow test, which he failed and then they would only feed him baby food and he fought back.

They wouldn't let me take him home, they insisted on rehab, until he could walk again, another disaster. My Wonderful Husband and I got a place a mile from the rehab facility (the RV Park where our camper was set-up, was on the opposite side of town) and I went there four or five times a day to take care of him. He refused the baby food, so I would take him for a ride in the wheelchair and we would go two-blocks away to a fast food place where he would happily eat two cheeseburgers, fries and a milkshake, never choking once. I would tell them to give him real food, but they could not, doctor's orders.

The combination of the virus and the forced immobility took its toll and his dementia got worse. He thought he was back in the service or in school and I would try to correct him. One day he said to me, "I'm happy, why are you sad?" That changed my perspective and I accepted HIS reality and we both had a great time after that. He even introduced me as his wife or his son George, occasionally, and I would say "Daaaddddd" and he would laugh. So, my Dad died of complications of a virus, the Parkinson's was the least of his problems.

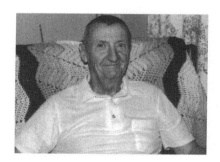

177

Meeting a President

My Dad was a weatherman in the Air Force and he usually worked in the control tower giving weather reports to pilots. He was stationed at Eglin AFB in the panhandle of Florida when I was born, two years later we went to Taegu AFB in South Korea, and two years after that to Andrews AFB, near Washington D.C, and home of Air Force One, the President's plane. He frequently gave reports to the pilots of Air Force One and I thought this was a really big deal, but to him, it was just another day at work.

When I was seven, I borrowed a neighbor kid's bigger bike. I could ride it, if I stood on the pedals, but I couldn't reach the seat. This bigger bike went much faster than my tiny one and faster was the excitement I was looking for. The street in front of our house was near the bottom end of a fairly steep hill. Our street didn't have much traffic on it, so all the kids in the neighborhood would take their toys (bikes, roller-skates and skateboards in summer and sleds and skis in the winter) and go up to the top of the hill and see how fast we could go on the way down.

There was a stop sign about halfway down, but we usually ignored it since there wasn't much traffic on that side street either. I was flying down the hill, having a grand time and woke up in the hospital. A UPS truck and I both tried to occupy the same intersection at the same time. I apparently flew over the handlebars of the bike and hit the side of the truck at full speed, headfirst. I don't remember what happened to the bike.

I got flown by helicopter to Walter Reed Military Hospital; with the top of my skull fractured in a nice L shape. I guess my head was pretty hard, it left a good-sized dent in the side of the truck, but it didn't cause any brain damage, though it was two days before I woke up with a bad headache.

It just so happened that former President Eisenhower was in the hospital at the same time, and since I was a serviceman's child with a big crack in my skull, someone decided that I should get to meet the former President. So, they wheeled me into his room and asked me if I knew who he was. I said no. Then they said, "This is the former President of the United States, Mr. Eisenhower." I said, "So what?" or "Who cares?" or something similar. Mom and Dad were completely embarrassed, but to me, he was just some old man in a hospital bed and besides, my head hurt.

I still have a fondness for UPS trucks, though I haven't run into any since then.

Now that I think about it, my Dad retired from the Air Force shortly after my Presidential blunder, I hope it wasn't a "forced" retirement.

179

Off We Go to Mexico

We took a trip to Mexico. The small border town of Algodones is just 25 miles away, so we park on the U.S.A. side and walk over. Once you cross into Mexico, the hawkers start their chants: "Need a Dentist?", "Need Glasses?", "Best prices on drugs" are standard ones. Then there are those who have a sense of humor: "Leather purses, made from real cows" or "Gold chains, almost free" and my favorite "Pretty dresses, for teenager like you". The sidewalks are uneven, the alleys are narrow and the hawkers sometimes get too close. I'm afraid of falling, so it's stressful. If I didn't have Parkinson's, I might enjoy it and look around, but I am in a hurry to get what I need and get back to the U.S.A.

Why go there? Algodones is filled with dentists, pharmacies and optical shops. You can buy leather goods, jewelry, liquor, pottery, clothes, hats, paintings, etc. You name it and Algodones probably has it and some of it is actually made in Mexico. You can buy all these items cheap, sometimes one tenth of what it would cost in the U.S.A.

I went to get medication for my Rosacea (red face) and $20 is a much better price than $85. The same Big Pharma makes the medicine; the only difference is the instructions are in Spanish.

First time visitors are shocked by the pharmacies; long shelves of medicines and signboards outside with prices. No prescriptions needed, but there are limits to how much you can bring back to the U.S.A., so we make several trips each year. Some folks go every few weeks.

Getting in takes minutes, getting out can take hours depending on the time of year. When my stepdaughter was here in February, it took 2 1/2 hours to get up to the gate. Today there was no line at all.

It was a hot and slow day in Algodones, even the watchdog was sleeping, but the hawkers were more gregarious than usual, so I didn't stop to look at purses or hats. I didn't even get a cinnamon roll; the bakery had closed for the summer.

I did go to the dentist and got some new glasses, and I'll tell you about those adventures in the next chapters. After my foreign excursion, what I really wanted was lunch and a nap (and I got both).

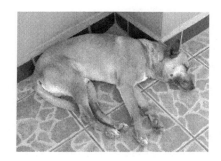

Oh, What Big Teeth You Have

While I was in Mexico, I went to the dentist for a cleaning. I have a lot of teeth in my mouth, thirty to be exact, and I don't have a big mouth (despite what my Parents said), so cleaning my teeth can be a challenge (many a dental tech has suggested I get a flip-top head, like is shown in a toothbrush ad). The Parkinson's makes it difficult for me to obey commands, my jaw and tongue have a mind of their own, so I need a dental tech with a sense of humor and who's not afraid of being bitten.

I'm not sure how many dentists occupy the small town of Algodones, but I'd guess it's close to 100. The dental offices are right next to each other. You can get everything from a simple cleaning to fillings, dentures, and even implants, all done at very reasonable prices, compared to U.S.A. I had a crown replaced several years ago for about $200.

Appointment times are subjective in Mexico, if your appointment is at 10 am, the dentist might not show up until 11 am, so you need to be a patient patient. I was lucky on this day, the dental assistant (probably a recent dental school grad) was there when I arrived and I only had to wait thirty minutes to be taken back to the room. She was very pretty with perfectly straight white teeth and long thick dark curly hair; it was like having a super-model clean my teeth. Too bad she wasn't a he; it would have been more fun for me.

The exam room looked just like every other dentist office

I have ever been to. They give you dark shades to wear, so the bright light doesn't hurt your eyes. They put Vasoline on your lips, so they don't crack from having your mouth wide open and they put a real towel under the paper one that clips around your neck, so your shirt doesn't get all wet. At my last visit to a U.S.A. dentist (which was 6 months ago), they did none of this.

The first thing she did was hang the suction tube thingy on my lip. It promptly fell off. She tried again and it fell off, so I reached my hand up and held it in place for the rest of the visit (you can't expect a dental tech to have three hands). Then she went to work, trying to wrangle the mirror and ultra-sonic wand around my moving tongue and lips. She kept asking me to open my mouth and to turn my head towards her. I didn't realize I was doing the opposite. She had a very difficult time reaching the back teeth, but managed somehow and I did NOT bite her, so it was a successful visit.

My guess is she will call in sick the next time I have an appointment. She wouldn't be the first. The reason I have thirty teeth is my teeth don't like to come out. The two I had extracted proved so difficult for the oral surgeons; they asked me to never come back!

Dental health is important if you have Parkinson's and taking care of your teeth can be challenging, so I go regularly for cleanings and exams. I use a power toothbrush and floss picks, since I have dexterity problems, but I still have all my fingers.

I Can See Clearly Now

When I was in Mexico, I got an eye exam and new glasses. Just like pharmacies and dentists, optical shops are prevalent in Algodones. I didn't need a change for distance, but I did need a change for close-up (easier to get new glasses than lengthen my arms). This particular change has nothing to do with Parkinson's, it, unfortunately means I'm just getting older. Darn, I can't blame it on the Parkinson's!

We got there early, and surprise, the Algodones Optical Shop was already open, so I had a chance to try on some new frames before the optician arrived at 8:30 am. They have frames of every size, shape and price range. I tried on a few and then got called into the exam room.

First he checked my pressures for glaucoma, they were good. He had me read the distance chart and began the usual "Which is clearer, lens A or B?" routine. Next he handed me the small print card, and my hands promptly began to shake. My tremors aren't bad, unless I am holding something in my hand with my elbow bent. I don't read books for this reason and I read the newspaper with it laying flat on the dining room table, so I don't have to hold it. Finally, he held the card for me and we got to where I could read the smallest type. Then he sent me out to pick out frames.

Picking out new frames is difficult, and I rely on my Wonderful Husband to choose what looks best. He hates this, but I tell him he sees me more than anyone, so I

184

only care if he likes them. I tried on dozens and we finally settled on a smaller frame than what I usually wear. I found a duplicate and gave both to the girl behind the counter (it was buy one, get one free).

The optician came back over, took some measurements and I was done. I decided to add some tint to one pair and asked to have my old glasses made into sunglasses. They said my new glasses would be ready in two hours, so I left and went to my dentist appointment.

When I was done at the dentist, all three were ready, my two new pair and new "old" sunglasses. They did some final adjustments, gave me a couple of cases and cleaning cloths and I wrote them a check for $50 (now you know why I go there). I checked out my new sunglasses and my brand new ones. I really like them, my Wonderful Husband did great!

We walked up the sidewalk where you line up to leave Mexico and headed back across the border.

Not a bad day, walked over at 8:15 am, got Rx, new glasses and teeth cleaned and walked back at 11:30 am.

But You Don't Shake

But you don't shake... I HATE those four words and every time I hear them, I want to scream!

I hear them often, from strangers, from cashiers, from salesmen; I have even heard it from doctors, nurses and pharmacists. They always come right after I say, "I have Parkinson's disease."

On the morning of June 9th, 2012, my Wonderful Husband and I drove 200 miles to San Diego to attend a Parkinson's Seminar hosted by the University of California at San Diego (UCSD) and the Parkinson's Association of San Diego. My built in GPS failed me, or I just couldn't remember what I saw on the map, I'm not sure which, but I took the wrong exit and got lost. I quickly realized my mistake and after several u-turns, found the signs and made it to the program, twenty minutes late. We signed in and found seats.

During the break, I met Karen & Sue, people I've met online through Twitter. I'm not sure which of us was more excited to meet the other, I guess it was a tie, but either way, I was glad to meet them in person.

I wandered around and introduced myself to some of the folks who were attending the seminar, told them about my Parkinson's Humor blog and gave them refrigerator magnets with the Parkinson's Humor web address on it. I even told a funny story or two.

Then it happened, those four words: "But you don't shake." I didn't scream, I didn't get mad, I just said, "You're right, I don't." I explained that tremors are the least of my problems now and are controlled fairly well by medications. He asked, "How long have you had PD?" I said twelve years. "Wow," he said, "How do you manage your symptoms so well?" I explained about charting my symptoms and a great relationship with my neurologist. A few others nearby, heard our conversation and asked me about charting. I explained it, told them I had written a story about it and gave them magnets with the Parkinson's Humor web address and told them how to find the story on my blog.

The seminar was very informative and afterwards I handed out a few more magnets and told a few people about my Parkinson's songs. I got to talk to several of the doctors who spoke at the seminar, and the best part was that none of the doctors said "but you don't shake" when I told them I have Parkinson's. That gives them an A+ in my book.

Shake and Bake

When I asked my Parkie friends to come up with things that were good about having Parkinson's, Angela, a young Mom said, "My kids say I can Shake N Bake like no one else." This sounded like a song to me, so I sat down and wrote one. The melody is *Billy Bayou*, an old country song and here are my lyrics.

I can no longer work at a bank
You don't want me driving a tank
I can't even walk the plank
But I can still Shake and Bake

Don't ask me to pour the wine
Or walk in a straight line
Some times I feel like I'm made of pine
But I can still Shake and Bake

My feet stumble when I walk
Some times you can't hear me talk
I have trouble putting on a sock
But I can still Shake and Bake

I have trouble dialing a phone
And scooping ice cream into a cone
My face looks like it's made out of stone
But I can still Shake and Bake

My cakes don't rise, they come out flat
When I flip eggs, they go splat
The kids give their meatballs to the cat
But I can still Shake and Bake

Shopping is difficult at the store
And I can barely mop the floor
Takes me forever to answer the door
But I can still Shake and Bake

I have trouble combing my hair
And getting up out of a chair
Putting on make-up might give you a scare
But I can still Shake and Bake

I can't sew a shirt that's been torn
Don't ask me to shuck the corn
Or change the diaper on a newborn
But I can still Shake and Bake
I can still Shake and Bake

Parkinson's: A Big Deal or Not

My Mom and Dad had strange senses of humor and liked to be silly but they were also very calm and mellow. Nothing was ever a big deal at our house. Nothing.

When Moomer went into labor with me, it was 2 pm and she was baking cookies for a Boy Scout meeting. She calmly finished baking the cookies, made Kool-Aid, arranged a sitter for the younger two kids, took the cookies and drinks to the den mother and asked her to keep the older two kids for awhile, then drove to the base (my Dad was in the Air Force), picked Dad up and went to the hospital. I was born at 4:44 pm. She said she had done it four times before, so it was no big deal.

It was the same with the accidents. When I was thirteen, I saw my brother get hit by a car and yelled, "David just got hit by a car." This was Moomer's very calm reply: "Go down the street and ask Mr. G. to come help me, call the ambulance and then come help me" as if she was reciting chores. She told Mr. G. what to do and then told me to calm down the driver (a boy my brother's age, sixteen).

The police and ambulances showed up and the trouble started. The car was in the county but David landed in the city, the centerline in the road was the divider. The police started arguing as to who had jurisdiction and who should do what. This got my Mom mad and in a drill sergeant voice, Moomer ordered Mr. G. and one of the paramedics to move David to our driveway (county) and then she told the city cops and ambulance to get the hell out of there! David had a broken leg but he was fine. No big deal.

Both Dad and Moomer liked to enter contests and often they won. The DJ on the radio would be whooping and hollering and Moomer would say, "That's nice." about the prize. Dad hit the lottery for several thousands of dollars and barely broke a smile. It was no big deal.

When my first husband died in a car crash when I was 23, my Parents said, "Everything will be fine." and pretended it was no big deal. When Moomer was diagnosed with terminal cancer a few months later, it was no big deal, she said, I'll always be with you. A few years later, I married my Wonderful Husband and everything WAS fine and Moomer is with me everyday in my heart, so, when I got diagnosed with Parkinson's at the age of 47, it really was NO BIG DEAL!

The ABC's of Parkinson's Handwriting

One of my earliest symptoms of Parkinson's was a change in my handwriting, though I didn't realize it at the time. Difficulty writing is the main thing I hate about having Parkinson's, and even though I joke about it in my songs, in reality, I don't find anything humorous about it.

The medical term for it is Micrographia and simply means small writing. Our letters tend to get smaller and smaller and closer together until we can no longer read it (heck, I don't think even a doctor could read mine). Add in some tremor and most of us just quit writing all together. I fall into this category.

Everything I have read has said the handwriting problems can't be fixed with therapy or even the DBS procedure, so I pretty much gave up hope of ever writing again, until now.

At the Parkinson's seminar I just attended in San Diego, I heard a speaker talk about reprogramming our brains to normal. She was discussing the idea of using large exaggerated movements to show our brains that small wasn't normal and she mentioned handwriting. She didn't elaborate, but I put on my thinking cap and decided to try an experiment.

If you have trouble writing, if it is getting tiny and cramped, I hope you will try this experiment with me.

Take a piece of paper and write the following: The quick brown fox jumped over the lazy sleeping dog 1 2 3 4 5 6

192

7 8 9 10 and sign your name.

Now, pretend that you are writing those exact same letters and numbers on a giant blackboard in the air, make the invisible letters as big as you possibly can, I did mine at least two-feet high.

Do the exercise a total of three times, I was holding the TV remote control in my hand, but you can use anything larger than a standard pen. If your arm gets too tired, just take a break and start again.

Now, take that same piece of paper and write the same thing as you did before and let me know if you see a difference (send me an email at yumabev@gmail.com). I was completely amazed at my results.

The improvement doesn't last, but why should it? Parkinson's is working against you 24-hours a day, so we have to keep fighting it. I found the improvement lasted a day or two, then the writing returned to small and illegible, but if I did the exercise again, or something similar, the improvement came back. I am thrilled to be able to write again and I hope you get similar results.

The quick brown fox jumped over the
lazy sleeping dog
1 2345678910
Beverly Ribaudo
Bun Rbd

The quick brown fox jumped
Over the lazy sleeping dog.

1 2 3 4 5 6 7 8 9 10

Beverly Ribaudo

Beverly Ribaudo

ParkinsonsHumor.com

194

Botched Recipes

Most everyone knows Parkinson's is caused by a loss of dopamine producing neurons in our brains, but most people don't know HOW the scientists get lab animals to have Parkinson's symptoms so they can be used for research (they don't go looking for animals with shaky paws). At the Parkinson's symposium hosted by the UCSD Movement Disorders Clinic and the Parkinson's Association of San Diego, I found out.

Back in the late 70's, the illegal drug culture spawned amateur home chemists who were cooking up concoctions in their kitchens, using available drugs (both over the counter and prescription), anything they could find in chemistry sets and under the kitchen sink. They would try their creations out on themselves and friends and if the desired high was achieved, they would make huge batches and sell it to others.

This is what happened in the San Francisco, California area back in 1982. One of these enterprising home chemists created something that he called new heroin and began selling it to local addicts. The chemical abbreviation for his creation was MPPP, which stands for words I can't even begin to pronounce. Unfortunately, one day, he messed up his recipe (he was probably high at the time) and ended up producing MPTP, another long unpronounceable chemical abbreviation, instead.

All of a sudden, addicts were showing up at area emergency rooms, looking like they had advanced Parkinson's. The onset was swift and irreversible, something had killed off most of their dopamine producing neurons and the public was warned about a dangerous new drug out on the streets. Eventually, the home laboratory was found and destroyed, but not before dozens of addicts were adversely affected.

A neurologist in the area, having been called in by the hospitals, realized the potential of this mistake and now, thanks to this botched recipe, scientists are able to give lab animals MPTP, or a variation of it, which causes them to have Parkinson's like symptoms, so they can be used for research.

The humor of this story: A stoned druggie screws up making a concoction to get himself stoned, ends up causing people to turn into stone and ultimately helps people with Parkinson's get un-stoned. You can't get much more ironic than that.

196

See How They Run

I went to three Parkinson's seminars (hosted by UC San Diego, the National Parkinson Foundation and the APDA) recently and the common theme was exercise is good for people with Parkinson's. This wasn't news to me, but I did learn the science behind it.

I heard some funny but serious quotes like, "Would you rather exercise one hour a day or be dead twenty-four?" and "Exercise can slow down the escalator to Parkinson's hell." Both of these are paraphrased because I've lost my short-term memory (if you find it, please return it).

So, here's the scoop. People are lazy and people with Parkinson's are worse. We can blame the laziness on the loss of dopamine, which not only helps control movement but is also one of the "feel good" chemicals in our brain. Since doing the things we used to do no longer "feels good," we Parkies tend to get lazier.

Researchers know this, so they gave rats, which are also lazy, Parkinson's symptoms by injecting them with MPTP or something similar. They then measured the movement abilities of the Parkie rats and compared them to non-Parkie rats. They took brain scans of both groups as well and carefully documented the results.

They then split the Parkie and non-Parkie rats into two groups: One group was allowed to do as they wished and the other group was forced to exercise by placing them on treadmills. It seems cruel to force them to walk or

197

run, but I guess that's why they use rats and not cute little puppies or kitties, most of us don't feel sorry for rats.

The results were exciting, the Parkie rats that were forced to exercise showed vast improvements over the Parkie rats that did nothing. The difference was noted not only in their movement ability, but changes were visible in the brain scans as well. The forced exercise didn't show much change in the non-Parkie rats (except maybe they were skinnier).

This proves that exercise is a very good thing, but you can't force people with Parkinson's to walk on treadmills, so we need to be motivated. Those quotes I mentioned above motivated me. I usually walk every morning, but now I have added walking on a treadmill to my daily routine and I feel better already. I shot video of my first day and my third day on the treadmill and saw an amazing difference.

So, my Parkie friends, don't be lazy rats, get up and exercise (and if you have a treadmill, use it).

Marching to a Different Beat

In the summer before I started junior high school, I decided to play clarinet. Why? Barbie. Barbie was my best friend and lived next door. She was a year older and had everything this twelve-year old did not. She was pretty, with thick wavy hair and straight teeth. I was still wearing clothing sized for first graders and she wore teen size clothes and needed a bra. Barbie played clarinet, so I wanted to play one, too.

The school held a band camp. The first thing they taught us was how to march, not how to play anything, just how to march. We had to take two steps for each yard line on a football field. I marked lines on my driveway with chalk and practiced until I could step off exactly eighteen-inches, even with my eyes closed. I never was a good clarinet player, but I was an excellent marcher. For years, I could accurately step off how many yards something was, until Parkinson's affected the way I walked and stole my built in yardstick.

In my ongoing effort to learn how to undo what Parkinson's has done to me, I attended a music therapy program at the Parkinson's conference in Irvine, California. The speaker stated that music could be used to improve your gait and help your brain re-learn how to walk normally. I was already doing treadmill exercises recommended by another speaker at the same conference, so I decided to add some music. I picked out some favorite tunes including some I used to play in my school band days (*Louie Louie* and *Tequila*) and

199

concentrated on walking to the beat. I noticed a big difference right away. My gait evened out and my arms began to swing like normal, plus it was fun thinking about those teenage years. I shot video to compare to the walking without music and there is definitely a difference.

I actually enjoy marching on my treadmill and the improvement in walking seems to be lasting all day. Maybe I'll get my built in ruler back. (Honey, where's the chalk?)

Hmm, I wonder what ever happened to that old clarinet.

PS This is the third story featured on the Michael J. Fox Foundation's website.

The Lineman

Several years ago, I went to a thrift store and saw a cute ladies t-shirt, it had "Lineman's Girl" and "Danger: High Voltage" on the front. I bought it and on the way home, I started thinking about Glen Campbell's big hit *Wichita Lineman*. The song starts out "I was a lineman for the county, and I drive the main roads." I started singing it but changed the first part to "I was a lineman for the county, until I got fired," then I started thinking just what a lineman might do to get fired and I came up with "touching the wrong wire." By the time I got home, about twenty minutes later, I had written "The Lineman." I made a funny costume and performed it at a talent show they held at the RV Park where I was living at the time. These are my lyrics:

I was a lineman for the county
'til I touched the wrong wire
When I hit the ground
My hair was still on fire
When they got me to the hospital
I was still throwing sparks
When I left three weeks later
I glowed in the dark

I think I'm doing pretty well
Though I have trouble when I walk
And if you get too close to me
You might just get a shock
I still feel the current in me
And I twinkle like a star

201

I can short out a pacemaker
or jump start your car

So if I seem a bit confused
Or my hair seems to shine
Its cuz this former lineman
Touched the wrong line
And if you see me shaking
If there's a gleam in my eye
If I wear crazy clothing
You know the reason why

The song always gets plenty of laughs and it's one of my favorites to perform.

Well, recently, I went to karaoke at a local restaurant and I decided to sing The Lineman. My hand was shaking as I held the microphone, but I didn't think anyone would notice or if they did, wouldn't care. I figured they'd just think I was nervous.

After I finished singing, a man came over to me and started telling me that he had been hit by lightning several years ago and that his hands still shook because of it. He then asked me how long I had been a lineman and how long ago I'd got zapped. He thought the story was true! I just laughed and said: "It's just a song inspired by a t-shirt I bought for 25 cents, I've never been a lineman or been electrocuted. The reason my hands shake is because I have Parkinson's."

He seemed disappointed.

Mind Over Matter, Gray Matter

People are always surprised when I answer black & white as my favorite color, not blue or pink or yellow. I like the definitive contrast, it's like yes or no, right or wrong, good or bad, night or day, hot or cold, ying or yang, humor or sadness.

I have more black & white shirts in my closet than any other color (zebra print, polka dots, stripes, floral, checks). You name it, I probably have it. In pants, jeans in various shades of blue dominate, but only because they match so well with the black & white shirts, however, I'm always on the lookout for a zebra print pair of jeans like Rod Stewart or Madonna might wear.

I have black & white print dishes; black & white accents on trash cans, file boxes, penholders, the paper shredder and the background for my Parkinson's Humor blog and Twitter pages.

I even have a black & white bedroom and it's one of a kind, because I made the quilt and curtains myself, from scraps of fabric left over from clothes I made over the years.

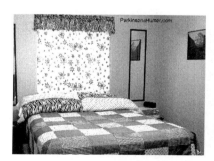

Then I got Parkinson's and there is nothing black & white about it. It's all gray. It's a disease of our brains or gray matter. No two people have the same symptoms or react the same way to medications; even the ribbon for Parkinson's is gray.

I guess it's fitting because everyone knows that if you mix black & white together, you get gray, but I wish at least one thing about Parkinson's could be black & white.

Maybe there is finally one thing about Parkinson's that I can say is black & white.

This book!

What a Difference a Year Makes!

2010 was not a good year for me, I felt awful for most of the year. I don't know if it was the Parkinson's or not. 2011 didn't start out well, either. My best friend Jeremy, whom I had known for thirty years, died on Jan 12th. I felt lost. My Wonderful Husband did his best, but even he couldn't fix this.

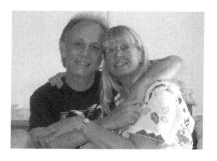

Jeremy and Me

March came and things changed for the better. I had written a song parody a few years earlier about the "snowbirds" leaving to go home for the summer and I decided to make a music video of the song and put it on YouTube. In April, the local NBC station (KYMA) contacts me and wants me to come on their morning show to talk about my funny song. I went and had a great time. During the breaks, everyone at the station was singing along to my song!

Then I saw an editorial in my local paper (*Yuma Sun*) about a Parkinson's seminar. I didn't know much about Parkinson's then, except that I had it. It sounded informative, so I went to the seminar and learned more about Parkinson's in two days than I had learned by having the disease for eleven years. A speaker said, "IF you are wide awake at 3 am and need someone to talk to, find a Parkinson's Chat Room, there will be other wide awake Parkies to chat with." I also found out about a local Parkinson's support group.

Within days, I was chatting with new friends from around the globe and they were laughing at my Parkinson's stories. One of them, Karyn from Australia, suggested I start a Parkinson's humor blog, so I did. I wrote my first story on July 17, 2011 and as of the writing of this book, I have written 100 more. Who'd of thought I had that much to say? I never, ever, expected so many people to read it (43,000 views from 119 different countries, so far). It amazes me everyday!

Now here it is, a year later and my life has completely changed. I have been on local TV three times; I started writing the Parkinson's Humor blog, which led me to writing this book. I have over 250 new Parkie Facebook friends, a couple dozen new Parkie chat room friends; a couple dozen more local Parkie friends and 500 Twitter Parkie friends and I still have my Wonderful Husband. To think it all started by reading a "Letter to the Editor".

I wonder what new adventures will come my way in the next year? Maybe Cat and I will actually get to meet Mr. Fox.

My Eight Year Journey to Diagnosis and The Letter

Several times in this book, I have mentioned how it took me eight years to get diagnosed with Parkinson's. The story isn't funny at all, but I think it is important, so I am putting it here, at the end of the book.

From 1999 to 2007, as I went from doctor to doctor trying to get an answer, each new one I saw would get my hopes up, he (or she) would say, "I know what's wrong with you." and then order the appropriate tests to prove their theory. Every time the tests came back negative, they would look at me; shake their heads and say, "I don't know."

Was it frustrating? Yes.

Did I often come home crying from the doctor's office? Yes.

Did I ever get depressed? No.

I was always upbeat and positive. How could that be?

It was simple; I realized early on that whatever I had wasn't fatal! If it was, I'd have been dead already and even though I got worse as the years went by, my quality of life didn't really change, until May of 2007.

I started to go downhill, fast. Every day I was worse than the day before. My regular doctor was on maternity leave and I didn't want to start all over with a new one so, I took matters into my own hands. I knew my problem had to be neurological, everything else had been ruled out.

I wrote a detailed letter explaining my symptoms and medical history, then got a listing of every neurologist within 500 miles from a medical board website. I started alphabetically and sent four or five letters a week and then waited for a response. When I got no replies, I sent a few more letters. This went on most of the summer.

I only heard back from ONE of them, Dr. Zonis, the last letter I sent. I almost didn't send the last few, I was so disappointed in getting no responses, but I had no choice. I was weeks away from being in a wheelchair. Yes, I was that bad.

Dr. Zonis called, said he knew what was wrong with me and asked me to come in the next day. His office was in the same town where I lived. I went, but I wasn't hopeful. All those years of "I don't know" had made me skeptical. When he said Parkinson's, I said, "Are you sure?" He said "Get this prescription filled, it's not very expensive, take three a day and if you don't feel better in a week, then I will be wrong, but I won't be wrong, you have Parkinson's."

He wasn't wrong! I felt better within 24 hours, and the change was unbelievable. I could actually move again! When I went back to see him a week later, I gave him a great big hug. Why? He didn't say "I Don't Know."

Here is the letter I wrote:

208

The Letter

July, Aug. 2007 (I updated the dates as I sent them out)

Hello,

I am looking for a neurologist who might be able to help me with my symptoms. I am slowly losing dexterity/coordination of my right hand/arm. I am a 47 year old right-handed white female in good health otherwise. This problem started about 8 years ago, shortly after I had a repetitive motion injury (never properly diagnosed) involving my right arm. The injury was to the area between my right shoulder blade and spine. Over the years I have had x-rays, chest CT, MRI from brain to t-spine, all kinds of blood tests, EKG, etc. with no help. I've seen 3 orthopedic docs, a back specialist, multiple internists and chiropractors. I have copies of most of the past reports. Here is my history:

Late 98', repetitive motion injury (quit job that caused injury) Dr. prescribed home physical therapy which I did for a year

Summer 99, went to work one day and could no longer double click my computer mouse with right index finger

Late '99, started having trouble writing

Early 2000, tremor started in right hand, by end of year I was doing most things left-handed because my tremor was so bad

2001, saw a bunch of Dr.'s and had lots of tests, nothing

2002-03, tremor worse, right hand/arm never feels relaxed

2004, decided to focus on tremor, more Dr.'s and tests, Diagnosis

209

of Essential Tremor, Dr. prescribed Propranolol

Some improvement with dexterity, though I still couldn't right click a mouse and my hand/arm still never feels relaxed

2005 to present: Tremor under control with minimum meds (Dr. lowered dose because my heart beat was too slow) Having more dexterity problems, trouble buttoning buttons, using scissors, tying bows, cutting meat (can't seem to coordinate both pushing down and going back and forth), writing (it takes forever to sign my name), brushing teeth (I hold the toothbrush still and move my head). It seems like I can do something one day and then the next I can't, and I never get it back. I do a lot left handed, but try to force myself to use the right one. My arm/hand never feels relaxed and my arm doesn't swing when I walk, it just hangs straight down. I have a tendency to hold my arm/hand like people do who are in vegetative state; I guess I'm trying to relax it. I have no numbness or tingling sensation and have not lost strength; I still pick up heavy items right handed. It seems like I feel best right after sleeping and it gets worse as the day goes on.

Also, a few years ago, I started to get a sensation occasionally in my right foot that my toes were being squeezed or curled under. This sensation occurs daily now and I don't wear tight shoes, in fact, when I get the sensation and look, they look the same as the left toes. I also seem to have trouble tapping my right foot and when I walk; my gait seems awkward, like my right leg is thudding down. I don't know if this is related to my right arm or not. I also startle easily and my husband says my reflexes are getting slower.

If you think you can help, please have someone contact me. I quit working several years ago when my husband retired, I just couldn't physically do my job anymore. I have no health insurance and we

210

earn a 'little too much' for me to qualify for Arizona's Medicaid. My husband gets Medicare. If you don't think you can help, maybe you could pass this on to someone who might.

Sincerely,

Beverly Ribaudo

The only things I left out of the medical history were the two neurologists I had already seen. I didn't want to prejudice a prospective new one.

The first neurologist I saw, in 2002, was my father's in Florida (Dad had Parkinson's); his exact words were "Don't waste my time, I can't help you, your problem isn't neurological."

The second neurologist I saw, in 2004, was in Colorado, and he diagnosed the Essential Tremor and point blank told me it was definitely NOT Parkinson's. He also said there was no need for follow-up visits. Many years later, I got copies of my medical records and I found this "Some rigidity present in right leg, Young Onset PD?" in his notes. Why did he say definitely not Parkinson's to me? I will never know, he died before I saw the notation.

What a price to pay. I had been unable to work since 2002 and IF either one of the first two neurologists I saw had got it right, my disability check would most likely be twice as much as it is.

The most interesting thing I've learned since my

211

diagnosis is the upper back pain was probably my first symptom, and yet, that pain seemed to cause the most confusion with the neurologist's I saw.

I got lucky with Dr. Zonis, not only did he get the diagnosis right, but he helped me get my disability claim approved. My point is, don't give up. There is a Dr. Zonis for everyone out there, keep searching.

I made and submitted a video of "The Letter" to the Neurological Film Festival in 2011. People with Parkinson's have seemed to like my entry; however, I don't think it went over well with the neurologists. Hmm, I wonder why?

THE END

About the Author

I hope you enjoyed my book, learned a few things and had a bunch of laughs. I'm Beverly (Bev) Ribaudo and I was finally diagnosed with Parkinson's disease at age 47, though my symptoms started in my late 30's. Humor comes naturally to me. A little disease like Parkinson's can't take it away. I have been married since 1985 to the most Wonderful Husband in the whole world. I like photography and I like to write my own song parodies. I combine both interests by creating music videos of my parodies. Due to laziness, I typed my name as YumaBev when I logged into a chat room and now I am known as Yuma Bev around the world, besides, everyone mispronounces my last name, including me. My Wonderful Husband says REE-bah-DOE and I say Rib-AH-doe. We don't worry about it; every family member says it differently.

Yuma (pronounced YOU-mah) Arizona is located in the southwest corner of the state, just north of Mexico and east of California. Yuma is a fairly good-sized city, we have three Wal-Marts, a Sam's Club, chain restaurants such as Olive Garden, Outback Steakhouse, Red Lobster and my favorite, Logan's Roadhouse and nice retail stores such as Macy's, Penney's and Dillard's. Yuma is about three hours from San Diego and Phoenix and about six hours from Las Vegas, and there's not much in between except desert and cacti!

Our winters are mild, with daytime highs usually near 70F; our summers are hot, with highs reaching 110+F.

213

We get very little rain and the sun shines 360+ days a year. Because of this fantastic winter weather, retirees from all over the U.S.A. and Canada flock to Yuma to spend their winters. The population quadruples in the winter, with many staying in RVs. In fact, being an RVer and looking for a place to spend the winter is how I ended up in Yuma.

Connect with me Online

Follow me on Twitter: @yumabev

Email address: yumabev@gmail.com

Parkinson's Humor blog: www.ParkinsonsHumor.com

The Parkinson's Humor YouTube Channel: www.youtube.com/parkinsonshumor

Facebook: Parkinson's Humor

Have a Happy Parkie Day!